# Military Mental Health Care

## Military Life

Military Life is a series of books for service members and their families who must deal with the significant yet often overlooked difficulties unique to life in the military. Each of the titles in the series is a comprehensive presentation of the problems that arise, solutions to these problems, and resources that are of much further help. The authors of these books—who are themselves military members and experienced writers—have personally faced these challenging situations, and understand the many complications that accompany them. This is the first stop for members of the military and their loved ones in search of information on navigating the complex world of military life.

*The Wounded Warrior Handbook: A Resource Guide for Returning Veterans* by Don Philpott and Janelle Hill (2008).

*The Military Marriage Manual: Tactics for Successful Relationships* by Janelle Hill, Cheryl Lawhorne, and Don Philpott (2010).

*Combat-Related Traumatic Brain Injury and PTSD: A Resource and Recovery Guide* by Cheryl Lawhorne and Don Philpott (2010).

*Special Needs Families in the Military: A Resource Guide* by Janelle Hill and Don Philpott (2010).

*Life After the Military: A Handbook for Transitioning Veterans* by Janelle Hill, Cheryl Lawhorne, and Don Philpott (2011).

*Military Mental Health Care: A Guide for Service Members, Veterans, Families, and Community* by Cheryl Lawhorne-Scott and Don Philpott (2013).

# Military Mental Health Care

## *A Guide for Service Members, Veterans, Families, and Community*

Cheryl Lawhorne-Scott
and Don Philpott

ROWMAN & LITTLEFIELD
*Lanham • Boulder • New York • London*

Published by Rowman & Littlefield
A wholly owned subsidiary of The Rowman & Littlefield Publishing Group, Inc.
4501 Forbes Boulevard, Suite 200, Lanham, Maryland 20706
www.rowman.com

Unit A, Whitacre Mews, 26-34 Stannary Street, London SE11 4AB


First paperback edition 2015



British Library Cataloguing in Publication Information Available

**Library of Congress Cataloging-in-Publication Data**

The hardback edition of this book was previously cataloged by the Library of Congress as follows:

Lawhorne-Scott, Cheryl, 1968-
Military mental health care : a guide for service members, veterans, families, and community / Cheryl Lawhorne and Don Philpott.
p. cm. — (Military life)
Includes bibliographical references and index.
1. Veterans—Mental health—United States—Handbooks, manuals, etc. 2. Veterans' families—United States—Handbooks, manuals, etc. 3. Soldiers—Mental health—United States—Handbooks, manuals, etc. 4. Psychology, Military—Handbooks, manuals, etc. I. Philpott, Don, 1946- II. Title.
UH629.3.L39 2013
355.3'45—dc23 2012034879

ISBN: 978-1-4422-2093-5 (cloth : alk. paper)
ISBN: 978-1-4422-5685-9 (pbk. : alk. paper)
ISBN: 978-1-4422-2094-2 (electronic)

™ The paper used in this publication meets the minimum requirements of American National Standard for Information Sciences—Permanence of Paper for Printed Library Materials, ANSI/NISO Z39.48-1992.

Printed in the United States of America

# Contents

# Foreword

*Stay Fit, Stay Strong, Stay Resilient!* This is not meant as merely a catch phrase or sound bite, but rather these words intend to serve as "a military standard" that both feeds and sustains our daily lifestyle!

Each of our service branches manages a resiliency program using the overarching model of Total Force Fitness (TFF). TFF is not a "How To" manual but rather a user-friendly, equal-opportunity framework to building a behavior, discipline, and level of fitness that sustains a lifestyle of resiliency. Our society has commonly narrowed how we view the word "fitness." Particularly in our military community, we tend to associate fitness with a level of physical ability. Truthfully, this is linear thinking. There is so much more to staying fit than running, pushups, and obstacle courses. Don't get me wrong, physical fitness is definitely an important piece, but there are other vital areas of fitness that repair and fuel the mind, body, and spirit. Nutritional, Behavioral, Psychological, Environmental, Financial, Social, and Spiritual are other critical fitness domains that serve as active ingredients to a holistic menu in our daily lifestyle. Said another way—we need all of these to preserve a total force that is and can remain totally fit.

While prevention will always be the ultimate goal, unfortunately in our line of work that is sometimes unavoidable. We define resiliency as having the ability to overcome adversity or setback, rebound from an incident and return to a renewed level of optimal performance. I think you will find that our various resiliency programs provide valuable resources in overcoming adversity and building resiliency in the mind, body, and spirit. As you read through these chapters, it will be evident that resiliency plays a critical role in all phases of the process from initial injury/incident through rehabilitation to sustaining optimality.

While many wounds, injuries, and illnesses or common setbacks warrant a medicinal solution, one of the things my wife Lisa and I enjoy about a TFF lifestyle is that at some point, opportunities arise for alternative or complementary methods of therapy and rehabilitation. Drug-free examples are yoga, meditation, acupuncture, peer-to-peer engagement, even a therapy dog to mention a few.

With twenty-five glorious years of marriage, sixteen household moves, deployments across the years, and injury and loss within our own family, she and I use our personal experiences to project how resiliency has largely and positively impacted our family successes and recovery throughout our career. We believe that an individual, family, unit, or organization that adopts a TFF lifestyle will consistently maintain a greater state of health, wholesomeness, stability, and readiness.

Lastly, Lisa and I always enjoy the opportunity such as this one, to recognize all military families for your longstanding commitment and remarkable service and sacrifice in defense of our nation!

Stay Fit! Stay Strong! Stay Resilient!

Bryan and Lisa Battaglia

Sgt. Major Bryan Battaglia is the Senior Enlisted Officer, Joint Chiefs of Staff at the Pentagon.

# Introduction

With tens of thousands of warriors returning from the wars in Iraq and Afghanistan every month, the Department of Defense (DoD) and Department of Veterans Affairs (VA) are almost overwhelmed by the task of providing adequate psychological and sociological support. One in three returning warriors has or is likely to develop serious mental health and/or psychological issues that make it difficult for them to adjust to a normal environment. As a result, many military marriages are ending in divorce, suicide rates among returning warriors are at record levels, and returning warriors make up a disproportionally high percentage of the unemployed and homeless. There is no single resource available that looks at all the problems these returning warriors and their families face. That is what the *Military Guide to Mental Health* aims to correct.

Mental health is how we think, feel, and behave. It helps determine how we adapt to a range of demands, relate to others, and make choices. Just like physical health, mental health is important at every stage of life and is essential to overall health.

This book has been written as an easy-to-use reference guide for injured service members as well as for their families and loved ones. There is a huge and growing amount of literature available from the military and others; there are scores of support organizations involved in this arena; and there are hundreds of websites offering information and help. All of these do a magnificent job in their respective areas but it can be a daunting task to pull together all this information, especially at a time of crisis. This information has been gathered from literally hundreds of these sources in the public domain.

A lot of the information included in this book comes from VA, the DoD, and all branches of the services. We acknowledge their cooperation and have made every effort to be as up to date and accurate as possible.

Our aim is to provide a comprehensive framework that will allow you to quickly access information that you need regarding medical treatment, rehabilitation, counseling, support, transition, and if needed, long-term care.

## The Extent of the Problem

Mental health problems are not a sign of weakness. The reality is that injuries, including psychological injuries, affect the strong and the brave just like everyone else. Some of the most successful officers and enlisted personnel have experienced these problems.

But stigma about mental health issues can be a huge barrier for people who need help. Finding the solution to your problem is a sign of strength and maturity. Getting assistance from others is sometimes the only way to solve something. For example, if you cannot scale a wall on your own and need comrades to do so, you use them! Knowing when and how to get help is actually part of military training.

Posttraumatic Stress Disorder (PTSD) is not the only serious problem that can occur after deployment. Watch out for signs of other conditions that are described in this book in yourself, your comrades, and family members.

War experiences and war zone stress reactions, especially those caused by personal loss, can lead a depressed person to think about hurting or killing him- or herself. If you or someone you know is feeling this way, take it seriously, and get help.

According to the National Consensus Statement on Mental Health Recovery, *"Mental health recovery is a journey of healing and transformation enabling a person with a mental health problem to live a meaningful life in a community of his or her choice while striving to achieve his or her full potential."*

In order to support the rehabilitation and recovery of every veteran with a mental illness, VA has identified recovery as a guiding principle for its entire mental health service delivery system. Recovery is a journey that involves developing hope, self-direction, empowerment, respect, and peer support.

# 1

# Traumatic Brain Injury

## What Is It?

A traumatic brain injury (TBI) is a blow or jolt to the head or a penetrating head injury that disrupts the function of the brain. Not all blows or jolts to the head result in a TBI. The severity of such an injury may range from "mild"—a brief change in mental status or consciousness—to "severe," an extended period of unconsciousness or amnesia after the injury. A TBI can result in short- or long-term problems with independent function.

## What Causes TBI?

The leading causes of TBI are:

- Bullets, fragments, blasts
- Falls
- Motor-vehicle traffic crashes
- Assaults

Blasts are a leading cause of TBI for active duty military personnel in war zones.

## Who Is at Highest Risk for TBI?

- Males are about 1.5 times as likely as females to sustain a TBI.
- Military duties increase the risk of sustaining a TBI.

The terms "concussion" and "mild TBI" (mTBI) are interchangeable. A TBI classified as moderate or severe can result in short-term or long-term problems with independent function. Most TBIs are mild, and those who sustain them usually recover completely within one to three months. In the military, the leading causes of TBI are given above.

## The Extent of the Problem

TBI is often referred to as the "signature wound" of the global war on terror. It's been reported that TBI could account for up to 50 percent of combat-related casualties and because of advances in trauma treatment, surgery, and rapid evacuation, many wounded warriors are now surviving what would just a few years ago have been fatal wounds. Many hundreds of thousands more service personnel are suffering from posttraumatic stress disorder (PTSD)—and in many cases, don't realize it (see below).

For wounded warriors with TBI there are now excellent treatment facilities such as the National Intrepid Center of Excellence on the Navy Campus at Bethesda, Maryland, next to the new Walter Reed National Military Medical Center. There is an ever-growing network of support groups—both official and unofficial—and a dedicated army of caregivers.

While it is advanced technology that has contributed to the survival rate of these warriors, it is also advanced technology that can assist them in coping and dealing with their challenges. Above all, however, these wounded warriors need care and loving attention. Thankfully, there are many willing to give it and to all of them, our grateful and continuing thanks.

One of the most difficult things about having a TBI is that people do not always have immediate symptoms. Also, sometimes the symptoms are present but not obvious. TBIs are common wounds in Operation Enduring Freedom (OEF)/Operation Iraqi Freedom (OIF) because of the frequent exposure to improvised explosive device (IED) blasts. The protective gear issued now is better than in previous wars. For instance, many who were exposed to blasts in Vietnam and in previous conflicts or wars did not survive.

The percentage of brain injury in Vietnam was 14 to 18 percent. Today, the survival rate is higher, but so is the brain-injury level. The newer complication is that while the body is protected, especially with the Kevlar helmets, the brain is literally shaken inside the protective brain sac. Blast injuries create extreme differences in air pressure, typically one thousand times greater than normal pressure, with a travel velocity of 1,600 feet per second. These shock waves that travel through the brain create small bubbles. Eventually these bubbles pop, leaving pockets or holes in the brain, similar to the holes found in baby Swiss cheese. Some authors have named this phenomenon "ghost shrapnel." If these bubbles occur inside blood vessels, they can form a blocked area, preventing oxygen from reaching that part of the brain, killing that section of the brain. Shock waves can also cause bruising and hemorrhaging in certain areas of the brain, killing surrounding cells. The level of damage is impacted by where you are in relation to the path of the shock waves, how you are situated in that path, the rate of the rise of pressure, and the length of the pressure wave, or the time frame.

Current reports indicate that approximately 20 percent of OEF/OIF vets have been diagnosed with TBI, and 40 percent of those diagnosed cases have received care. Walter Reed Army Medical Center reported that 31 percent of the people admitted there between early 2003 through mid-2005 had some level of TBI. It is thought that there are many more cases of service members with brain injuries that have yet to be diagnosed. While the percentages do not look greatly different than those from Vietnam, the level and type of brain injury is quite different. Many service members are deployed multiple times within theater, greatly increasing their chance of getting more than one concussion.

## TBI Surveillance

The Defense and Veterans Brain Injury Center (DVBIC) track the numbers of service members who sustain a TBI in order to improve care delivery within the Department of Defense (DoD) and Department of Veterans Affairs (VA). Understanding the scope of the problem in our warrior population is essential to determine the ideal level of response at the local, regional and national level. Specifically, improving the accuracy of statistical information helps to direct existing medical assets, develop and expand educational and clinical resources, and allows for deeper appreciation of the issue by providers and family members alike.

DVBIC began collecting surveillance data on service members who sustained a TBI in OEF/OIF in 2003. Data was obtained from DVBIC affiliated sites at military treatment facilities, VA hospitals, and civilian rehabilitation centers. In 2007, DVBIC was designated as the Office of Responsibility for the consolidation of all TBI-related incidences and prevalence information for the DoD. Today, DVBIC continues to receive new data on a monthly basis from all service branches.

## How Does It Manifest Itself?

*Symptoms of Mild TBI (mTBI) or Concussion*

- Headaches
- Dizziness
- Excessive fatigue (tiredness)

- Concentration problems
- Forgetting things (memory problems)
- Irritability
- Balance problems
- Vision change
- Sleep disturbance

One of the most common observations reported by families of service members originally not diagnosed with mTBI is that upon return from deployment, they "have changed." Classic neurological and cognitive symptoms of mTBI that should be recognized and discussed with medical professionals include:

- Reduced reaction time
- Decision-making difficulties
- Decreased memory and forgetfulness
- Attention and concentration difficulties
- Confused about recent events
- Repeating of thoughts and questions
- Personality changes
- Impulsiveness
- Anger
- Sadness
- Depression
- Nervousness
- Changes in sleep patterns

Service members often overlook the symptoms of mTBI because they don't think that they are serious issues; they don't want to admit to the injury to their peers; or they don't have time to attend to these symptoms due to the fatigue and stress of a wartime environment.

While these symptoms may seem subtle to you and not obvious to others, many service members do not want to mention these symptoms to others. This is a mistake.

Awareness of the symptoms is critical for you and your family because even a doctor may not be able to recognize the subtle changes at the initial visit. Acknowledging these injuries is no longer considered a weakness, but rather a sign of strength and personal responsibility.

You must be your own advocate by knowing the symptoms for all types of brain injuries and seeking immediate medical advice if you experience any of them. The sooner these injuries are diagnosed, the more effective the treatment, and the sooner you'll be able to regain lost abilities and adapt to changes.

### SUDDEN FEELINGS OF ANXIETY OR PANIC

These are a common part of traumatic stress reactions, and include sensations of your heart pounding and feeling lightheaded or "spacey" (often due to rapid breathing). If this happens, remember that:

These reactions are not dangerous. If you had them while exercising, they would not worry you.

It is the addition of inaccurate frightening thoughts (e.g., I'm going to die, I'm having a heart attack, I will lose control) that makes them especially upsetting.

Slowing down your breathing may help.

The sensations will pass soon and you can still "go about your business" after they decrease.

Each time you think in these positive ways about your arousal / anxious reactions, you will be helping them to happen less frequently. Practice will make it easier to cope.

### FEELING LIKE THE TRAUMA IS HAPPENING AGAIN ("FLASHBACKS")

Keep your eyes open. Look around you and notice where you are.

Talk to yourself. Remind yourself where you are, what year you're in, and that you are safe.

Trauma happened in the past, and you are in the present.

- Get up and move around. Have a drink of water, and wash your hands.
- Call someone you trust and tell that person what's been happening.
- Remind yourself that this is quite common traumatic stress reaction.
- Tell your counselor or doctor what happened to you.

### TRAUMA-RELATED DREAMS AND NIGHTMARES

- If you awaken from a nightmare in a "panic," remind yourself that you are reacting to a dream and that's why you are anxious / aroused . . . and not because there is real danger now.
- Consider getting up out of bed, "regrouping," and orienting yourself.
- Engage in a pleasant, calming activity (e.g., listen to soothing music).
- Talk to someone if possible.
- Talk to your doctor about your nightmares; certain medications can be helpful.

### DIFFICULTY FALLING OR STAYING ASLEEP

- Keep to a regular bedtime schedule.
- Avoid strenuous exercise within a few hours of going to bed.

- Avoid using your sleeping area for anything other than sleeping or sexual intimacies.
- Avoid alcohol, tobacco, and caffeine. These harm your ability to sleep.
- Do not lie in bed thinking or worrying. Get up and enjoy something soothing or pleasant; reading a calming book, drink a glass of warm milk, do a quiet hobby.

IRRITABILITY, ANGER, AND RAGE

- Take a "time out" to cool off or to think things over. Walk away from the situation.
- Get in the habit of using daily exercise as a friend. Exercise reduces body tension and helps get the "anger out" in a positive and productive way.
- Remember that anger doesn't work. It actually increases your stress and can cause health problems.
- Talk to your counselor or doctor about your anger. Take classes in "anger management."
- If you blow up at your family or friend, find time as soon as you are able to talk to them about it. Let them know how you feel, and what you are doing to cope with your reactions.

DIFFICULTY CONCENTRATING

- Slow down. Give yourself time to "focus" on what it is you need to learn or do.
- Write things down. Making "to do" lists may be helpful.
- Break task down into small do-able "chunks."
- Plan a realistic number of events or tasks for each day.
- Perhaps you may be depressed; many who are do have trouble concentrating. Again, this is something you can discuss with your counselor, doctor, or someone close to you.

HAVING DIFFICULTY FEELING OR EXPRESSING POSITIVE EMOTIONS

- Remember that this is a common reaction to trauma, that you are not doing this on purpose, and that you should not feel guilty for something you do not want to happen and cannot control.
- Make sure to regularly participate in activities that you enjoy or used to enjoy. Sometimes, these activities can rekindle feelings of pleasure.
- Take steps to communicate caring to loved ones in little ways: write a card, leave a small gift, phone and say hello.

- Experiment with these ways of coping to find which ones are helpful to you. Practice them, because, like other skills, they work better with practice. Talk to your counselor or doctor about them. Reach out to people in VA, Vet Centers, your family, and your community who can help. You're not alone.

## What Are the Treatment Options?

*Recovery from TBI*

- Get plenty of sleep at night and rest during the day.
- Return to normal activities gradually, not all at once.
- Until you are better, avoid activities that can lead to a second brain injury such as contact or recreational sports. Remember to use helmets and safety belts to decrease your risk of having a second brain injury.
- Don't drink alcohol; it may slow your brain recovery and it puts you at risk of further injury.
- If it's harder to remember things, write them down.
- If you find you are losing important items, begin putting them in the same place all the time.
- If you are easily distracted or having difficulty concentrating, try doing only one thing at a time in a quiet, nondistracting environment.
- If you feel irritable, then remove yourself from the situation that's irritating you or use relaxation techniques to help manage the situation. Irritability is worse when you are tired, so rest will help.
- Be patient! Healing from a brain injury takes time.

Symptoms of mTBI or concussion often resolve within hours to days and almost always improve over one to three months. However, if symptoms persist without improvement, medical treatment should be sought.

Unlike a severe or even moderate TBI, a concussion or mTBI may not be readily identified. Recognizing the importance of early detection, the DoD and VA have established system-wide screening and assessment procedures to identify concussion/mTBI in service members and veterans at the soonest opportunity and through multiple points of care.

Screening for concussion/mTBI involves a quick evaluation of possible exposure to a traumatic event including injuries that may occur during deployment, leave, or even civilian life following active duty. Clinicians work to establish if there was an alteration of consciousness (AOC) associated with the injury or traumatic event, and if the event resulted in any neurologic changes or symptoms.

Because concussion/mTBI is not always recognized in the combat setting, screening of active duty service members also occurs through post-deployment health assessments (PDHA). Four questions that are adapted from the Brief Traumatic Brain Injury Survey (BTBIS) appear on the PDHA. Positive responses on all four questions should prompt a clinician interview to more fully evaluate for concussion/mTBI.

## Understanding the Recovery Process

Knowing how recovery happens puts you in more control of the recovery process.

- Recovery is an ongoing, daily, gradual process. It doesn't happen through being suddenly "cured."
- Some amount of continuing reactions is normal and reflects a normal body and mind. Healing doesn't mean forgetting traumatic war experiences or having no emotional pain when thinking about them.
- Healing may mean fewer symptoms and less disturbing symptoms, greater confidence in ability to cope with your memories and reactions, and improved ability to manage emotions.

## Coping with Traumatic Stress Reactions: Ways that DON'T Help

- Using drugs and alcohol as ways to reduce anxiety or relax, stop thinking about war experiences, or go to sleep. Alcohol and drug use cause more problems than they cure.
- Keeping away from other people. Social isolation means loss of support, friendship, and closeness with others, and more time to worry or feel hopeless and alone.
- Dropping out of pleasurable or recreational activities. This leads to less opportunity to feel good and feel a sense of achievement.
- Using anger to control others. Anger helps keep other people away and may keep bad emotions away temporarily, but it also keeps away positive connections and help from loved ones.
- Trying to constantly avoid people, places, or thoughts that are reminders of the traumatic event. Avoidance of thinking about trauma or seeking treatment doesn't keep away distress, and it prevents progress on coping with stress reactions.
- Working all the time to try and avoid distressing memories of the trauma (the "workaholic").

## Coping with Traumatic Stress Reactions: Ways that CAN Help

There are many ways you can cope with posttraumatic stress. Here are some things you can do if you have any of the following symptoms:

UNWANTED, DISTRESSING MEMORIES, IMAGES, OR THOUGHTS

- Remind yourself that they are just that—memories.
- Remind yourself that it's natural to have some sorts of memories of the event(s).
- Talk to someone you trust about them.
- Remember that although reminders of trauma can feel overwhelming, they often lessen over time.

## Classification and Natural History of Traumatic Brain Injuries (TBI) Severity

Many patients and clinicians assume that the terms mild, moderate, and severe TBI refer to the severity of symptoms associated with the injury. In fact these terms refer to the nature of the injury itself. Here are the accepted definitions:

- Mild traumatic brain injury is defined as a loss or alteration of consciousness shorter than thirty minutes, posttraumatic amnesia shorter than twenty-four hours, focal neurologic deficits that may or may not be transient, and/or Glasgow Coma Score (GCS) of 13 to 15.
- Moderate traumatic brain injuries entail loss of consciousness longer than thirty minutes, posttraumatic amnesia longer than twenty-four hours, and an initial GCS 9 to 12.
- Severe brain injuries entail all of the moderate criteria listed above, but with a GCS less than 9.

### *Mild TBI*

About 80 percent of all TBIs in the civilian population are mTBIs. The primary causes of TBIs in the civilian population are falls, motor vehicle accidents, being struck by an object, and assaults. Immediately subsequent to the initial insult, 80 to 100 percent of patients with mTBI will experience one or more symptoms related to their injury, such as headache, dizziness, insomnia, impaired memory, and/or lowered tolerance for noise and light. In most cases of mTBI the patient returns to his or her previous level of function within three to six months, and it is important to reassure patients about this fact. However, some 10 to 15 percent of patients may go on to develop chronic postconcussive symptoms. These symptoms can be grouped into three categories: somatic (headache, tinnitus, insomnia, etc.), cognitive (memory, attention, and concentration difficulties), and emotional/behavioral (irritability, depression, anxiety, behavioral dyscontrol). Patients who have experienced mTBI are also at increased risk for psychiatric disorders compared to the general population, including depression and PTSD.

In the military population, the emerging picture is somewhat different. The primary causes of TBI in veterans of Iraq and Afghanistan are blasts, blast plus motor vehicle accidents (MVAs), MVAs alone, and gunshot wounds. Exposure to blasts is unlike other causes of mTBI and may produce different symptoms and natural history. For example, veterans seem to experience the postconcussive symptoms described above for longer than the civilian population; some studies show most will still have residual symptoms eighteen to twenty-four months after the injury. In addition, many veterans have multiple medical problems. The comorbidity of PTSD, history of mTBI, chronic pain, and substance abuse is common and may complicate recovery from any single diagnosis. Given these special considerations, it is especially important to reassure veterans that their symptoms are time-limited and, with appropriate treatment and healthy behaviors, likely to improve.

### *Moderate and Severe TBI*

Patients with moderate and severe brain injuries often have focal deficits and, occasionally, profound brain damage. However, it should be noted that the severity of the initial injury does not correlate in a linear fashion with the severity of the brain damage, and that some of these patients can make remarkable recoveries. They may need ongoing cognitive and vocational rehabilitation, case management, and pharmacological intervention to return to their highest level of function.

## Diagnosis

The diagnosis of TBI, associated postconcussive symptoms, and other comorbidities such as PTSD presents unique challenges for diagnosticians. No screening instruments available can reliably make the diagnosis; the gold standard remains an interview by a skilled clinician. The current VA screening tool is intended to initiate the evaluation process, not to definitively make a diagnosis.

Details of the original injury can be elusive. Patients with moderate and severe brain injuries often, though not always, have unequivocal evidence of the relationship of their symptoms to their injury. Patients who have experienced mTBI can be more difficult to diagnose. The brevity of the initial alteration of consciousness may cause the initial injury to go unnoticed and the patient may present sometime after the original injury when details are unclear. Another factor is that these injuries can occur in chaotic circumstances, such as combat, and may be ignored in the heat of events. Clinicians may be presented with vague concerns and little relevant detail about the original injury; whenever possible, clinicians and patients should attempt to obtain supporting documentation. At minimum clinicians should elicit as detailed an injury history as possible.

Once the injury history has been established, the patient's course of recovery and remaining postconcussive symptoms should be documented. Because of the considerable symptom overlap between postconcussive symptoms and symptoms of many psychiatric and neurologic disorders, this process can be challenging. Clinicians should have a low threshold to consult available expertise when making these diagnoses.

Patients with TBI often meet criteria for PTSD on screening instruments for TBI and vice versa. Some of these positive screens may represent false positives, but many OEF/OIF veterans have experienced a mild traumatic brain injury AND ALSO have PTSD related to their combat experience.

## Treatment

To manage this new injury profile, VA has initiated the polytrauma system of care, which treats patients with traumatic brain injury who also have experienced musculoskeletal, neurologic, and psychological trauma. Many of the most severely injured polytrauma patients are already receiving treatment at one of the four Polytrauma Rehabilitation Centers or one of the twenty-one Polytrauma Network Sites. Patients with milder injuries may present for treatment at other locales, including their local VAs or in their communities. Regardless of where a patient engages in treatment initially, there is no "wrong door" for treatment and VA is working to ensure that any barriers to access are minimized.

Randomized controlled trials have demonstrated that education for the patient and family early in the course of recovery can improve outcomes in patients with TBI and help to prevent the development of other psychological problems. Unfortunately, for reasons outlined above, many patients and their families do not receive education early in the course of illness and may require intervention after symptoms have become well established. Currently, VA encourages a recovery message when prognosis is discussed, and inclusion of the family in treatment planning. Treatments for PTSD, mTBI and other comorbidities should be symptom-focused and evidence based in concurrence with current practice guidelines (available at *VA/DoD Clinical Practice Guidelines*). For example, early data shows that the treatments that have worked well in veterans with PTSD alone, such as cognitive processing therapy and prolonged exposure or SSRIs can also work well for veterans who have suffered a mTBI as well as emotional trauma. Memory aids can also be useful in this population. Patients can also benefit from occupational rehabilitation and case management, depending on the severity of their injuries. Patients should be referred to consultants, such as neurologists, neuropsychologists, and substance abuse or other specialized treatment as needed.

Given the complexity of treatment plans for these veterans, careful collaboration and coordination of care between all providers is a critical element of treatment success. VA is exploring ways to enhance this collaboration, particularly in more community-based outpatient clinics and more rural environments.

### *Concussions or Mild Traumatic Brain Injury (mTBI)*

Explosions that produce dangerous blast waves of high pressure rattle your brain inside your skull and can cause mTBI. Helmets cannot protect against this type of impact. In fact, 60 to 80 percent of service members who have injuries from some form of blast may have TBI.

Symptoms associated with mTBI (or concussion) can parallel those of PTSD but also include:

- Headaches or dizziness
- Vision problems
- Emotional problems, such as impatience or impulsiveness
- Trouble concentrating, making decisions, or thinking logically
- Trouble remembering things, amnesia
- Lower tolerance for lights and noise

Know that PTSD is often associated with these other conditions. However, there are effective treatments for all of these problems.

Symptoms of mTBI or concussion often resolve within hours to days and almost always improve over one to three months. However, if symptoms persist without improvement, medical treatment should be sought.

TBI is a significant health issue that affects service members and veterans during times of both peace and war. The high rate of TBI and blast-related concussion events resulting from current combat operations directly impacts the health and safety of individual service members and subsequently the level of unit readiness and troop retention. The impacts of TBI are felt within each branch of the service and throughout both the DoD and VA health care systems.

In VA, TBI has become a major focus secondary to recognition of the need for increased resources to provide health care and vocational retraining for individuals with a diagnosis of TBI, as they transition to veteran status. Veterans may sustain TBIs throughout their lifespan, with the largest increase as the veterans enter into their seventies and eighties; these injuries are often due to falls and result in high levels of disability.

Active duty and reserve service members are at increased risk for sustaining a TBI compared to their civilian peers. This is a result of several factors, including the specific demographics of the military; in general, young men between the ages of eighteen to twenty-four are at greatest risk for TBI. Many operational and training activities which are routine in the military are physically demanding and even potentially dangerous. Military service members are increasingly deployed to areas where they are at risk for experiencing blast exposures from IEDs, suicide bombers, land mines, mortar rounds, rocket-propelled grenades, and so on. These and other combat-related activities put our military-service members at increased risk for sustaining a TBI.

Although recent attention has been intensively focused on combat-related TBI, it should be noted that TBI is not uncommon even in garrison and occurs during unusual daily activities; service members enjoy exciting leisure activities: they ride motorcycles, climb mountains, and parachute from planes for recreation. In addition, physical training is an integral part of the active duty service members' everyday life. These activities are expected for our service members and contribute to a positive quality of life, but these activities can also increase risk for TBI.

The following sections delve deeper into issues of TBI and the military. Topics aim to increase awareness of the unique issues which contribute to TBI in the military and what is being done to support the care and recovery of combat wounded troops and veterans with TBI.

TBI occurs from a sudden blow or jolt to the head. Brain injury often occurs during some type of trauma, such as an accident, blast, or a fall. Often when people refer to TBI, they are mistakenly talking about the symptoms that occur following a TBI. Actually, a TBI is the injury, not the symptoms.

### *How Serious Is My Injury?*

A TBI is basically the same thing as a concussion. A TBI can be mild, moderate, or severe. These terms tell you the nature of the injury itself. They do not tell you what symptoms you may have or how severe the symptoms will be.

A TBI can occur even when there is no direct contact to the head. For example, when a person suffers whiplash, the brain may be shaken within the skull. This damage can cause bleeding between the brain and skull. Bruises can form where the brain hits the skull. Like bruises on other parts of the body, for mild injuries these will heal with time.

About 80 percent of all TBIs in civilians are mild (mTBI). Most people who have a mTBI will be back to normal by three months without any special treatment. Even patients with moderate or severe TBI can make remarkable recoveries.

The length of time that a person is unconscious (knocked out) is one way to measure how severe the injury was. If you weren't knocked out at all or if you were out for less than thirty minutes, your TBI was most likely minor or mild. If you were knocked out for more than thirty minutes but less than six hours, your TBI was most likely moderate.

### *What Are the Common Symptoms Following a TBI?*

Symptoms that result from TBI are known as postconcussion syndrome (PCS). Few people will have all of the symptoms, but even one or two of the symptoms can be unpleasant. PCS makes it hard to work, get along at home, or relax. In the days, weeks, and months following a TBI the most common symptoms are:

PHYSICAL

- headache
- feeling dizzy
- being tired
- trouble sleeping
- vision problems
- feeling bothered by noise and light

COGNITIVE (MENTAL)

- memory problems
- trouble staying focused
- poor judgment and acting without thinking
- being slowed down
- trouble putting thoughts into words

EMOTIONAL (FEELINGS)

- depression
- anger outbursts and quick to anger
- anxiety (fear, worry, or feeling nervous)
- personality changes

These symptoms are part of the normal process of getting better. They are not signs of lasting brain damage. These symptoms are to be expected and are not a cause for concern or worry. More serious symptoms include severe forms of those listed above, decreased response to standard treatments, and seizures.

## *Assessment*

**Table 1.1 Some of the Various Techniques That Can be Used to Determine Degree of Exposure and the Relevant Measures to be Adopted**

| *Trauma Exposure Measures* | *Target Group* | *Format* | *# of Items* | *Time to Administer (Minutes)* | *Assesses DSM-IV Criterion A* |
|---|---|---|---|---|---|
| Combat Exposure Scale (CES) | Adult | Self-Report | 7 | 5 | No |
| Evaluation of Lifetime Stressors (ELS) | Adult | Self-Report and Interview | 56 | 60–360 | Yes |
| Life Stressor Checklist-Revised (LSC-R) | Adult | Self-Report | 30 | 15–30 | Yes |
| National Women's Study Event History | Adult | Interview | 17 | 15–30 | A-1 only |
| Potential Stressful Events Interview (PSEI) | Adult | Interview | 62 | 120 | Yes |
| Stressful Life Events Screening Questionnaire (SLESQ) | Adult | Self-Report | 13 | 10–15 | No |
| Trauma Assessment for Adults (TAA) | Adult | Self-Report and Interview | 17 | 10–15 | A-1 only |
| Trauma History Screen (THS) | Adult | Self-Report | 13 | 2–5 | Yes |
| Trauma History Questionnaire (THQ) | Adult | Self-Report | 24 | 10–15 | A-1 only |
| Traumatic Events Questionnaire (TEQ) | Adult | Self-Report | 13 | 5 | A-1 only |
| Traumatic Life Events Questionnaire (TLEQ) | Adult | Self-Report | 25 | 10–15 | A-1 only |
| Trauma History Questionnaire (THQ) | Adult | Self-Report | 24 | 10–15 | Yes |
| | Adult | Interview | 9 | 5–30 | A-1 only |

## How Can Family and Friends Assist in the Healing Process?

The primary source of support is likely to be the soldier's family. We know from veterans of the Vietnam War that there can be a risk of disengagement from family at the time of return from a war zone. We also know that emerging problems with acute stress disorder (ASD) and PTSD can wreak havoc with the competency and comfort the returning soldier experiences as a partner and parent. While the returning soldier clearly needs the clinician's attention and concern, that help can be extended to include his or her family as well. Support for the veteran and family can increase the potential for the veteran's smooth immediate or eventual reintegration back into family life and reduce the likelihood of future more damaging problems.

If the veteran is living at home, the clinician can meet with the family and assess with them their strengths and challenges and identify any potential risks. Family and clinician can work together to identify goals and develop a treatment plan to support the family's reorganization and return to stability in coordination with the veteran's work on his or her own personal treatment goals.

If one or both partners are identifying high tension or levels of disagreement, or the clinician is observing that their goals are markedly incompatible, then issues related to safety need to be assessed and plans might need to be made that support safety for all family members. Couples who have experienced domestic violence and/or infidelity are at particularly high risk and in need of more immediate support. When couples can be offered a safe forum for discussing, negotiating, and possibly resolving conflicts, that kind of clinical support can potentially help to reduce the intensity of the feelings that can become dangerous for a family. Even support for issues to be addressed by separating couples can be critically valuable, especially if children are involved and the parents anticipate future coparenting.

## Resources Available

- CDC's National Center for Injury Prevention and Control: www.cdc.gov/ncipc/tbi/TBI.htm
- National Institute of Neurological Disorders and Stroke (NINDS) Traumatic Brain Injury Information Page: www.ninds.nih.gov/disorders/tbi/tbi.htm
- Traumatic Brain Injury National Resource Center: www.pmr.vcu.edu
- Brainline (DVBIC-sponsored): www.brainline.org
- Brain Injury Association of America: www.biausa.org

# 2

# Stress

Recognizing the stresses military life and multiple deployments put on families, the services are stepping up their efforts to help their members strengthen their family relationships and avoid the divorce courts.

A full range of outreach programs—from support groups for spouses of deployed troops to weekend retreats for military couples—aims to help military families endure the hardships that military life often imposes.

## What Is It?

During missions there are multiple stages and types of conflict. Throughout an operation, these stages can overlap depending on the location and mission of assigned forces. Each form of conflict may contribute to different forms or expressions of stress. It is therefore valuable to determine precisely the nature and duration of exposures for returning troops.

### *Predeployment Phase*

During predeployment phase military members face uncertainty and worry. Deployment orders change routinely, sometimes with multiple revisions of deadlines and locations. Service members worry about the safety of themselves as well as their family members.

They struggle to ensure that finances, health care, childcare, and pets all will be managed in their absence. In the current climate, deploying service members may have additional concerns about terrorist activities in the United States during the period of deployment. Predeployment can be extremely stressful on single parents, reserve forces, and military members who have not previously deployed. It is often difficult during this phase to determine the difference between reasonable anxiety and an excessive reaction or the development or recurrence of psychiatric illness.

*Deployment Phase*

The deployment phase carries many additional pressures. The stress of traditional, high-intensity warfare leads to fear and uncertainty. Operational plans change constantly; knowledge of enemy capabilities is unclear; equipment breaks down; and logistical supply lines are uncertain. Combatants face the threat of their own death or injury and also witness the death, wounding, and disfigurement of their companions, enemy forces, and civilians.

During this heightened physiologic state, the high level of emotion and the intensity of sensory exposure may lead to heightened levels of arousal, attempts to avoid emotion, and intrusive recollections of events. The novelty of the situation may also contribute to symptoms of dissociation. The severity and duration of symptoms varies among individuals. This phase of combat is highly conducive to acute stress disorder and posttraumatic stress disorder in military members.

## Types of Conflict

Low-intensity combat is typical during peacemaking and peacekeeping missions.

Fear of death or injury is less imminent, but chronically present. Some troops may intermittently encounter the exposures found in high-intensity combat. The majority experience chronic strain of deployment: family separation, heat, cold, harsh living conditions, extremely long duty hours with little respite, minimal communication with the outside world, and boredom. These strains can result in the development of adjustment disorders, mood disorders, anxiety disorders, and exacerbations of personality disorders. Some members with predisposing factors may develop psychotic disorders. Depending on the availability of substances of abuse, abuse or dependence disorders may develop, recur, or worsen (Jones 1995a).

Terrorist activities and guerilla warfare tactics, such as car bombings, remotely detonated explosives, and mortar attacks lead to chronic strain and anxiety. Psychologically this can contribute to service members questioning their purpose, as well as negative attributions about the importance and need for the sacrifices encountered. Coupled with other exposures, exposure during this phase may exacerbate illness or delay recovery. Many of the veterans from prior wars have focused on their discontent associated with sacrifice and loss in a mission viewed as unpopular and unsuccessful.

In a highly armed nation such as Iraq or Afghanistan, US troops cannot be certain whether an innocent appearing civilian may be carrying a firearm, an explosive, or a remote-detonation device. Rules of engagement are altered regularly by command in response to political and tactical requirements.

When an individual or a vehicle challenges a roadblock or security checkpoint, a delay in the use of force may result in friendly forces injuries. A premature response may result in the unnecessary death of civilians. Such conditions create chronic strain, particularly when split-second decisions may undergo retrospective analyses to determine their appropriateness (Jones 1995b).

Friendly-fire events are among the most tragic. In the current military environment of high-technology communication, command, and control, there is a much lower risk of such occurrences. When they take place it is usually when there are failures of communication between allied forces. To date, no major events have occurred during this campaign, but have occurred during Operation Enduring Freedom, the war in Afghanistan. Similar to terrorist and guerilla acts, friendly-fire incidents (either by those responsible for or those who experienced the act) also lead to negative attributions about purpose of mission and specifically about the failure of leadership in preventing such outcomes. Friendly-fire incidents can be more difficult for service members to cognitively reconstruct, leading to less opportunity for integration and potential greater traumatic impact.

Clinical assessment must not assume that the experiences of all service members coming out of Iraq or Afghanistan are identical. Exposure to military conflict can be of a variety of types and intensities. A careful assessment should ensure that there is a complete understanding of all predeployment and deployment happenings. As a military patient may be reluctant to share details of his or her experiences early on with an unfamiliar provider, a thoughtful and detailed accounting of experiences will likely require the time to develop a trusting therapeutic relationship. As is clear from the information presented above, a service member's emotional response to wartime exposures is determined by the specific experiences, but equally important is the context in which these experiences are encountered and the meanings they hold.

## The Extent of the Problem

The psychological, social, and psychiatric toll of war can be immediate, acute, and chronic. These time intervals reflect periods of adaptation to severe war-zone stressors that are framed by different individual, contextual, and cultural features (and unique additional demands), which are important to appreciate whenever a veteran of war presents clinically.

The immediate interval refers to psychological reactions and functional impairment that occur in the war zone during battle or while exposed to other severe stressors during the war. The immediate response to severe stressors in the war zone has had many different labels over many centuries (e.g., combat fatigue); the label "combat stress reaction" is used most often currently.

However, this is somewhat a misnomer. As we discuss below, direct combat exposure is not the only source of severe stress in a war zone such as Iraq. The term "war-zone stress reaction" carries more meaning and is less stigmatizing to service personnel who have difficulties as a result of experiences other than direct life-threat from combat. Generally, we also want to underscore to clinicians that being fired upon is only one of the many different severe stressors of the war zone.

In the war zone, service personnel are taxed physically and emotionally in ways that are unprecedented for them. Although trained and prepared through physical conditioning, practice, and various methods of building crucial unit cohesion and buddy-based support, inevitably, war-zone experiences create demands and tax service personnel and unit morale in shocking ways. In addition, the pure physical demands of war-zone activities should not be underestimated, especially the behavioral and emotional effects of circulating norepinephrine, epinephrine, and cortisol (stress hormones), which sustain the body's alarm reaction (jitteriness, hyper vigilance, sleep disruption, appetite suppression, etc.). In battle, service personnel are taxed purposely so that they can retain their fighting edge. In addition, alertness, hyper vigilance, narrowed attention span, and so forth are features that have obvious survival value. Enlisted service personnel, noncommissioned officers, and officers are trained to identify the signs of normal "battle fatigue" as well as the signs of severe war-zone stress reactions that may incapacitate military personnel. However, the boundary line between "normal" and "pathological" response to the extreme demands of battle is fuzzy at best.

Officers routinely use postbattle "debriefing" to allow service personnel to vent and share their emotional reactions. The theory is that this will enhance morale and cohesion and reduce "battle fatigue."

Even if service personnel manifest clear and unequivocal signs of severe war-zone stress reactions that affect their capacity to carry out their responsibilities, attempts are made to restore them to duty as quickly as possible by providing rest, nourishment, and opportunities to share their experiences, as close to their units as possible. The guiding principal is known as Proximity-Immediacy-Expectancy-Simplicity ("PIES"). Early intervention is provided close to their unit, as soon as possible. They are told that their experience is normal and they can expect to return to their unit shortly. They are also provided simple interventions to counteract "fatigue" (e.g., "three hots and a cot"). The point here is that service personnel who experience severe war-zone stress reactions likely will have received some sort of special care. On the other hand, it is without question stigmatizing to share fear and doubt and to reveal signs of reduced capacity. This is especially true in the modern, all volunteer, military with many service personnel looking to advance their careers. Thus, it is entirely possible that some veterans who present at VA medical centers will have suffered silently and may still feel a great need to not show vulnerability because of shame.

The formal features of severe incapacitating war-zone stress reactions are restlessness, psychomotor deficiencies, withdrawal, increased sympathetic nervous system activity, stuttering, confusion, nausea, vomiting, and severe suspiciousness and distrust. However, because they will vary considerably in the form and course of their decompensation as a result of exposure to extreme stress, military personnel are prone to use a functional definition of combat fatigue casualty. For commanders, the defining feature is that the soldier ceases to function militarily as a combatant, and acts in a manner that endangers himself or herself and his or her fellow service members. If this kind of severe response occurs, the soldier may be evacuated from the battle area. Finally, clinicians should keep in mind that most combatants are young and that it is during the late teens and early twenties when vulnerable individuals with family histories of psychopathology (or other diatheses) are at greatest risk for psychological decompensation prompted by the stress of war. As a result, a very small number of veterans of the Iraq War may present with stress-induced severe mental illness.

For service personnel who may be in a war zone for protracted periods of time, with ongoing risks and hazards, the acute adaptation interval spans the period from the point at which the soldier is objectively safe and free from exposure to severe stressors to approximately one month after return to the United States, which corresponds to the one-month interval during which acute stress disorder (ASD) may be diagnosed according to the *Diagnostic and Statistical Manual of Mental Disorders* (DSM-IV). This distinction is made so that a period of adaptation can be identified that allows clinicians to discern how a soldier is doing psychologically when given a chance to recover naturally and receive rest and respite from severe stressors.

Otherwise, diagnostic labels used to identify transient distress or impairment may be unnecessarily pathologizing, stigmatizing, and inappropriate because they are confounded by ongoing exposure to war-zone demands and ongoing immediate stress reactions. Typically, in the acute phase, they are in their garrison (in the United States or overseas) or serving a security or infrastructure building role after hostilities have ceased.

The symptoms of ASD include three dissociative symptoms (Cluster B), one reexperiencing symptom (Cluster C), marked avoidance (Cluster D), marked anxiety or increased arousal (Cluster E), and evidence of significant distress or impairment (Cluster F). The diagnosis of ASD requires that the individual has experienced at least three of the following: (a) a subjective sense of numbing or detachment, (b) reduced awareness of one's surroundings, (c) derealization, (d) depersonalization, or (e) dissociative amnesia. The disturbance must last for a minimum of two days and a maximum of four weeks (Cluster G), after which time a diagnosis of posttraumatic stress disorder (PTSD) should be considered (see below).

Research has shown that that there is little empirical justification for the requirement of three dissociation symptoms. Accordingly, experts in the field advocate for consistency between the diagnostic criteria for ASD and PTSD because many individuals fail to meet diagnostic criteria for ASD but ultimately meet criteria for PTSD despite the fact that their symptoms remain unchanged.

Unfortunately, there have been insufficient longitudinal studies of adaptation to severe war-zone stressors. On the other hand, there is a wealth of research on the temporal course of posttraumatic reactions in a variety of other traumatic contexts (e.g., sexual assault, motor vehicle accidents). These studies have revealed that the normative response to trauma is to experience a range of ASD symptoms initially with the majority of these reactions remitting in the following months. Generalizing from this, it is safe to assume that although acute stress reactions are very common after exposure to severe trauma in war, the majority who initially display distress will naturally adapt and recover normal functioning during the following months. Thus, it is particularly important not to not be unduly pathologizing about initial distress or even the presence of ASD.

The chronic phase of adjustment to war is well known to VA clinicians; it is the burden of war manifested across the lifespan. It is important to note that psychosocial adaptation to war, over time, is not linear and continuous. For example, most are not debilitated in the immediate impact phase, but they are nevertheless at risk for chronic mental health problems implicated by experiences during battle. Also, although ASD is an excellent predictor of chronic PTSD, it is not a necessary precondition for chronic impairment—there is sufficient evidence to support the notion of delayed PTSD. Furthermore, the majority of people who develop PTSD did not meet the full diagnostic criteria for ASD beforehand. It is also important to appreciate that psychosocial and psychiatric disturbance implicated by war-zone exposure waxes and wanes across the lifespan (e.g., relative to life demands, exposure to critical reminders of war experiences, etc.). PTSD is one of many different ways a veteran can manifest chronic postwar adjustment difficulties. Veterans are also at risk for depression, substance abuse, aggressive behavior problems, and the spectrum of severe mental illnesses precipitated by the stress of war.

### *Stress and Marriage*

Specific service-by-service statistics about divorce rates within the military weren't available, but the rates for the Army give a snapshot of what are believed to be a military-wide trend.

Army officials reported 10,477 divorces among the active-duty force in fiscal 2004, a number that has climbed steadily over the past five years. In fiscal 2003, the Army reported fewer than 7,500 divorces; in 2002, just over 7,000, and in 2001, about 5,600.

During the past two years, the divorce rate has been higher among Army officers than their enlisted counterparts, reversing the previous trend, officials said. In fiscal 2003, the Army reported almost 1,900 divorces among its fifty-six thousand married officers. The following year, that number jumped to more than 3,300—an increase of almost 1,500.

These statistics reflect a general trend in American society, Army Chaplain (Col.) Glen Bloomstrom, director of ministry initiatives for the Army's Office of the Chief of Chaplains pointed out. Forty-five to 50 percent of all first marriages end in divorce nationwide, he said, and the failure rate is even higher for second marriages: a whopping 60 to 70 percent.

Divorce rates run even higher in specific occupations, particularly those that expose people to traumatic events and danger, as well as heavy responsibilities and public scrutiny, Army officials noted. Police officers, for example, face a divorce rate averaging between 66 and 75 percent, they said.

Despite the nationwide trends, Bloomstrom was quick to point out that the numbers represent far more than just statistics. "These are people we're talking about," he said. "When a marriage ends, it's the end of a dream."

The toll goes beyond the human side, and affects military operations as well, he said. Service members in happy marriages tend to be more focused on their jobs and less likely to become disciplinary problems, Bloomstrom said. They're also more likely to remain in the military.

To help reverse the statistics, the services have introduced new programs and pumped up existing ones, offered through their family support, chaplain, and mental health counseling networks.

For example, the Army's offerings include:

- The new Deployment Cycle Support Program, which includes briefings for soldiers on how their absence and return may affect their family relationships and how they can cope with the inevitable changes;

- A family-support group system that provides both practical and emotional support for spouses of deployed soldiers;
- The Building Strong and Ready Families Program, a two-day program that helps couples develop better communication skills, reinforced by a weekend retreat;
- The Strong Bonds marriage-education program that focuses specifically on issues that affect Reserve and National Guard couples; and The Pick a Partner program that helps single soldiers make wise decisions when they choose mates.

The Army is not alone in offering programs to help its families survive the rigors of deployments and strengthen their relationships in the process.

The Marine Corps' Prevention and Relationship Enhancement Program is a two-day workshop that teaches couples how to manage conflict, solve problems, communicate effectively and preserve and enhance their commitment and friendship, Marine officials said.

Participants begin the program by taking a marriage survey, developed by a retired Navy chaplain, to help them evaluate their relationship and identify problems before they become serious. The four top problems generally involve communication, children and parenting, money, and sexual intimacy, according to a Navy chaplain involved in the program.

The Marine Corps program focused on what the chaplain calls "the mother lode of all issues" that can affect marriages: communication. "If you don't have good communication skills, you can't talk about the rest of the issues," he said.

The Navy has a similar program in its Marriage Enrichment Retreat. This weekend getaway is designed to give Navy couples the tools they need to help strengthen their marriages, according to Rachelle Logan, public affairs director for Navy Installations Command.

Participants begin the weekend session by getting a profile of their personalities, then attending sessions on marital communication, personality and family dynamics, and problems associated with military separation, Logan said.

While the Air Force does not have service-wide marital support programs, Air Force officials said individual bases offer a wide variety of programs to support military families and help them through separations, deployments, and the stresses relating to them.

Bloomstrom said he's optimistic about the emphasis the military services are putting on programs for married service members.

The goal, he said, is to help couples recognize and address danger signs before they escalate.

Another objective is to help military couples get more satisfaction out of their marriages by injecting a healthy dose of "fun and friendship" that he said builds up their "emotional bank account."

"We're talking about investing in the relationship in the good times," he said. "That way, when you have to make a withdrawal—as you do during a deployment—you still have enough left in the bank to cover it."

## How Does It Manifest Itself?

*Coping with Stress*

Physical signs of a stress response include:

- Rapid heartbeat
- Headaches
- Stomachaches
- Muscle tension

Emotional signs of stress can be both positive and upsetting:

- Excitement, frustration, anxiety
- Exhilaration, nervousness, anger
- Joy, discouragement

*Managing Stress*

Stress management involves relaxing as well as tensing up. Relaxation actually is a part of the normal stress response.

When faced with life's challenges, people not only tense up to react rapidly and forcefully, but they also become calm in order to think clearly and act with control.

Techniques for managing stress include:

- Body and mental relaxation
- Positive thinking
- Problem solving
- Anger control
- Time management
- Exercise
- Responsible assertiveness
- Interpersonal communication

Physical benefits of managing stress include:

- Better sleep, energy, strength, and mobility
- Reduced tension, pain, blood pressure, heart problems, and infectious illnesses

Emotional benefits of managing stress include:

- Increased quality of life and well-being
- Reduced anxiety, depression, and irritability

### *Quick Stress-Reduction Techniques*

When you feel stressed, your breathing becomes fast and shallow and your muscles get tense. You can interrupt the stress response by:

- Slowing your breathing and taking deep, slow breaths from your belly.
- Relaxing your muscles (e.g., by tensing and releasing muscles throughout your body).

## MENTAL REFRAMING

Everyone has a stream of private thoughts running through their minds. This is called *self-talk*. These thoughts reflect your beliefs and attitudes about the world, other people, and yourself, and they may be adding to your stress. To interrupt the automatic thought process:

Become aware: monitor your thoughts and self-talk.

Recognize that thoughts cause feelings and motivate behavior. There is rarely a direct link between the stressful situation and your response. In fact, it's usually not the event or situation that leads to a stress reaction; *it's your interpretation of the event or situation* that causes you to respond in various ways.

The sequence of events that leads to feelings and behaviors in response to stressors is called the "*ABCs*":

You experience the *Activating* event.

Your *Beliefs* about the event lead to an interpretation of the event.

Your interpretation of the event either increases or decreases the stress you feel—the *Consequences*.

So:

*A* (*A*ctivating event) + *B* (*B*eliefs) = *C* (*C*onsequences)

Check your thoughts and self-talk for these stress-promoting thinking patterns:

- *All-or-nothing thinking*: judging things as being all good or all bad usually based on a single factor.
- *Exaggeration*: blowing the negative consequences of a situation or event way out of proportion.
- *Overgeneralization*: drawing conclusions about your whole life based on the negative outcome of a single incident.
- *Mind-reading*: believing you know what another person or group of people is thinking about you (usually bad) when you have no evidence.

Challenge your negative thoughts and self-talk by asking yourself whether there is evidence to support the way you are perceiving the situation.

Replace negative or stressful self-talk with more positive, useful, and realistic self-talk.

*Example*: While on leave, you decide to take the bus to go visit your family and get stuck in traffic due to road construction. Change *negative self-talk* ("This will take forever. I will never get home. Why does this always happen to me?") to *positive and useful self-talk* ("I'm glad they are fixing this road. I can take this time to relax and listen to some music I enjoy.")

### CONTROLLING THE SOURCE OF STRESS BY SOLVING PROBLEMS

Take action over stressors that you can control (your own habits, behavior, environment, relationships) by using the problem-solving process:

- Step 1: Define the problem.
- Step 2: Set a goal (for example, what would you like to see happen?).
- Step 3: Brainstorm possible solutions.
- Step 4: Evaluate the pros and cons of various possible solutions.
- Step 5: Choose the best solution (weigh the pros and cons).
- Step 6: Make a plan to implement the solution and try it!
- Step 7: Assess how well it went.
- Step 8: If the first solution doesn't work, try others.

### IF A SOURCE OF STRESS IS BEYOND YOUR CONTROL

Try an activity to distract or soothe yourself:

- Listen to music.
- Get together with a friend.
- Read a good book or watch a movie.
- Engage in physical exercise.

- Consider spiritual activity such as prayer.
- Perform yoga.
- Use humor (jokes or funny movies).
- Meditate.
- Take a nap.
- Write in a journal or diary.
- Take a hot bath or shower.
- Help others in need.
- Express your stress creatively.
- Take a "mental holiday."

#### PLAN FOR FUTURE STRESSFUL EVENTS

*Create* a personalized "Stress Toolkit" by making a list of coping strategies that work for you when you're stressed, including deep breathing, muscle relaxation, and activities that you find soothing.

- *Visualize* potential future stressful situations.
- *Determine* if you will have some control in the situation.
- *Decide* how you will use the problem-solving process to reduce stressors.
- *Plan* to use various helpful activities to reduce the stress response.
- *Remember* to include friends and family for support.

## What Are the Treatment Options?

### *Are There Effective Treatments for ASD?*

#### COGNITIVE-BEHAVIORAL INTERVENTIONS

At present, cognitive-behavioral interventions during the acute aftermath of trauma exposure have yielded the most consistently positive results in terms of preventing subsequent posttraumatic psychopathology. Four out of five randomized clinical trials (RCTs) related to early cognitive-behavioral interventions during the acute aftermath of trauma found that the cognitive-behavioral therapy (CBT) group experienced a greater reduction of PTSD symptoms than comparison groups. One of the RCTs did not find this to be true. The study by Brom, Kleber, and Hofman (1993) found that all three active conditions (desensitization, hypnotherapy, and psychodynamic therapy) yielded equal improvement relative to the waitlist control group. However, the Brom et al. study lacked a treatment adherence measure so it is unclear whether the CBT intervention was implemented in a standardized manner relative to other studies of CBT.

A different controlled (but not randomized) comparison of a CBT versus an assessment-only course of action in the acute phase posttrauma found fewer PTSD symptoms in the CBT group at a five-and-a-half-month follow-up.

Bryant et al. (1998) have conducted the only studies that specifically assessed and treated ASD. They have shown that a brief cognitive-behavioral treatment may not only ameliorate ASD, but it may also prevent the subsequent development of PTSD. Approximately ten days after exposure to an MVA, industrial accident, or nonsexual assault, Bryant et al. randomly assigned those with ASD to five individual, one-and-a-half-hour sessions of either a cognitive-behavioral treatment or a supportive counseling control condition. They found that fewer CBT subjects met criteria for PTSD posttreatment six months later. In the 1999 study, Bryant et al. compared two different individual CBT approaches (prolonged exposure plus anxiety management and prolonged exposure alone) to a supportive counseling intervention. They found that both CBT groups showed significantly greater reductions in PTSD symptom severity compared to the supportive counseling group.

#### PSYCHOLOGICAL DEBRIEFING?

Psychological debriefing is an early intervention that was originally developed for rescue workers that has been more widely applied in the acute aftermath of potentially traumatic events. However, RCTs of debriefing have yielded inconsistent findings in terms of its efficacy. A review of the literature on debriefing RCTs concluded that there is little evidence to support the continued use of debriefing with acutely traumatized individuals. Mitchell and Everly (2000), the originators of the debriefing model, have made the cogent argument that most of the debriefing RCTs to date have studied only one component (debriefing) of the longer-term and more comprehensive Critical Incident Stress Management model. It is possible that this more comprehensive intervention would prove efficacious, but to date no RCTs have been conducted using the full intervention.

### How Can Family and Friends Assist in the Healing Process?

With deployment comes change. Knowing what to expect and how to deal with changes can make homecoming more enjoyable and less stressful. Below are some hints you might find helpful.

*Expectations for Service Personnel*

- You may miss the excitement of the deployment for a while.
- Some things may have changed while you were gone.
- Face-to-face communication may be hard at first.
- Sexual closeness may also be awkward at first.
- Children have grown and may be different in many ways.
- Roles may have changed to manage basic household chores.
- Spouses may have become more independent and learned new coping skills.
- Spouses may have new friends and support systems.
- You may have changed in your outlook and priorities in life.
- You may want to talk about what you saw and did. Others may seem not to want to listen. Or you may not want to talk about it when others keep asking.

*Expectations for Spouses*

Your partner

- May have changed.
- Used to the open spaces of the field, may feel closed in.
- May be overwhelmed by noise and confusion of home life.
- May be on a different schedule of sleeping and eating (jet lag).
- May wonder if they still fit into the family.
- May want to take back all the responsibilities they had before they left.
- May feel hurt when young children are slow to hug them.

*What Children May Feel*

- Babies less than one year old may not know you and may cry when held.
- Toddlers (one to three years) may hide from you and be slow to come to you.
- Preschoolers (three to five years) may feel guilty over the separation and be scared.
- School age (six to twelve years) children may want a lot of your time and attention.
- Teenagers (thirteen to eighteen years) may be moody and may appear not to care.
- Any age child may feel guilty about not living up to your standards.
- Some may fear your return ("Wait until mommy/daddy gets home!").
- Some may feel torn by loyalties to the spouse who remained.

## Resources Available

- TRS Point of Contact Information: www.tricare.mil/reserve/reserve select/index.cfm
- TRICARE: www.tricare.osd.mil
- TRICARE For Life (TFL): www.tricare.mil/tfl
- TRICARE Health Benefits Advisors/Beneficiary Counselor and Assistance Coordinators (BCAC) Locator: www.tricare.mil/bcacdcao/

POSTTRAUMATIC STRESS DISORDER (PTSD) RESOURCES

- DoD Mental Health Self-Assessment Program: www.pdhealth.mil/militarypathways.asp
- National Center for Posttraumatic Stress Disorder (PTSD): www.ptsd.va.gov
- Ameriforce Deployment Guide: www.ameriforce.net/deployment/
- Courage to Care: www.usuhs.mil/psy/courage.html
- Returning Reservists Resources: www.usuhs.mil/psy/GuardReserve ReentryWorkplace.pdf
- Continued Health Care Benefit Program (CHCBP): www.humana-military.com/chcbp/main.htm
- CHCBP enrollment application: www.humana-military.com/chcbp/pdf/dd2837.pdf
- VA Home Page: www.va.gov/
- VA Health Care Enrollment Resources: www.1010ez.med.va.gov/sec/vha/1010ez/
- VA Eligibility: www.va.gov/healtheligibility/
- TRICARE Dental Program: www.tricare.mil/dental
- TRICARE Retiree Dental Program: www.trdp.org/

# 3

# Posttraumatic Stress Disorder

PTSD can occur after you have been through a traumatic event. Professionals do not know why it occurs in some people and not others. But we do know PTSD is treatable.

### Symptoms of PTSD

- Startling easily
- Feeling as though a certain event is happening again
- Having nightmares of terrifying events and night sweats
- Feeling distant from those you previously felt close to
- A feeling of numbness
- Feeling more aggressive or even violent
- Chronic intrusive recalling of events
- Feelings of guilt, "Why did I live and someone else died?"
- Feelings of despair
- Suffering addiction
- Contemplating suicide
- Difficulty trusting
- Feeling anxious
- Experiencing sleep problems
- Reliving the traumatic event(s) with flashbacks; these may include triggers like sounds, smells, feelings, and loud noises
- Avoiding the anniversary of the event
- Avoiding social events or places that spark memories

*Reexperiencing*

Bad memories of a traumatic event can come back at any time. You may feel the same terror and horror you did when the event took place.

Sometimes there's a trigger: a sound, sight, or smell that causes you to relive the event.

*Avoidance and Numbing*

People with PTSD often go to great lengths to avoid things that might remind them of the traumatic event they endured. They also may shut themselves off emotionally in order to protect themselves from feeling pain and fear.

*Hypervigilance or Increased Arousal*

Those suffering from PTSD may operate on "high alert" at all times, often have very short fuses, and startle easily.

*How Likely Are You to Get PTSD?*

It depends on many factors, such as

- How severe the trauma was
- If you were injured
- The intensity of your reaction to the trauma
- Whether someone you were close to died or was injured
- How much your own life was in danger
- How much you felt you could not control things
- How much help and support you got following the event

## Steps to Solving the Problem and Getting Help

PTSD is a treatable condition. If you think you have PTSD, or just some of its reactions or symptoms (such as nightmares or racing thoughts), it's important to let your doctor or even a chaplain know. These people can help you set up other appointments as needed.

There are several steps to addressing PTSD:

- Assessment: having a professional evaluate you with a full interview; educating yourself and your family about PTSD, its symptoms, and how it can affect your life.
- Some antidepressants can relieve symptoms of PTSD. These medications do not treat the underlying cause, yet do provide some symptom relief.

- CBT generally seeks to balance your thinking and help you express and cope with your emotions about the traumatic experience.

There are different types of therapy but in most you will learn

- How the problem affects you and others
- Goal setting about ways to improve your life
- New coping skills
- How to accept your thoughts and feelings, and strategies to deal with them

You are encouraged to meet with several therapists before choosing one. Finding a therapist involves learning

- What kinds of treatment each therapist offers
- What you can expect from the treatment and the therapist
- What the therapist expects of you

In 2000, the American Psychiatric Association revised the PTSD diagnostic criteria in the fourth edition of its *Diagnostic and Statistical Manual of Mental Disorders* (DSM-IV-TR). The diagnostic criteria (Criterion A–F) are specified below.

Diagnostic criteria for PTSD include a history of exposure to a traumatic event meeting two criteria and symptoms from each of three symptom clusters: intrusive recollections, avoidant/numbing symptoms, and hyperarousal symptoms. The fifth criterion concerns duration of symptoms and a sixth assesses functioning.

### CRITERION A: STRESSOR

The person has been exposed to a traumatic event in which both of the following have been present:

1. The person has experienced, witnessed, or been confronted with an event or events that involve actual or threatened death or serious injury, or a threat to the physical integrity of oneself or others.
2. The person's response involved intense fear, helplessness, or horror. Note: in children, it may be expressed instead by disorganized or agitated behavior.

### CRITERION B: INTRUSIVE RECOLLECTION

The traumatic event is persistently reexperienced in at least one of the following ways:

1. Recurrent and intrusive distressing recollections of the event, including images, thoughts, or perceptions. Note: in young children, repetitive play may occur in which themes or aspects of the trauma are expressed.
2. Recurrent distressing dreams of the event. Note: in children, there may be frightening dreams without recognizable content.
3. Acting or feeling as if the traumatic event were recurring (includes a sense of reliving the experience, illusions, hallucinations, and dissociative flashback episodes, including those that occur upon awakening or when intoxicated). Note: in children, trauma-specific reenactment may occur.
4. Intense psychological distress at exposure to internal or external cues that symbolize or resemble an aspect of the traumatic event.
5. Physiologic reactivity upon exposure to internal or external cues that symbolize or resemble an aspect of the traumatic event.

### CRITERION C: AVOIDANT/NUMBING

Persistent avoidance of stimuli associated with the trauma and numbing of general responsiveness (not present before the trauma), as indicated by at least three of the following:

1. Efforts to avoid thoughts, feelings, or conversations associated with the trauma
2. Efforts to avoid activities, places, or people that arouse recollections of the trauma
3. Inability to recall an important aspect of the trauma
4. Markedly diminished interest or participation in significant activities
5. Feeling of detachment or estrangement from others
6. Restricted range of affect (e.g., unable to have loving feelings)
7. Sense of foreshortened future (e.g., does not expect to have a career, marriage, children, or a normal life span)

### CRITERION D: HYPERAROUSAL

Persistent symptoms of increasing arousal (not present before the trauma), indicated by at least two of the following:

1. Difficulty falling or staying asleep
2. Irritability or outbursts of anger
3. Difficulty concentrating
4. Hypervigilance
5. Exaggerated startle response

CRITERION E: DURATION

Duration of the disturbance (symptoms in B, C, and D) is more than one month.

CRITERION F: FUNCTIONAL SIGNIFICANCE

The disturbance causes clinically significant distress or impairment in social, occupational, or other important areas of functioning.

Specify if

- Acute: if duration of symptoms is less than three months
- Chronic: if duration of symptoms is three months or more

Specify if

- With or without delay onset: onset of symptoms at least six months after the stressor

### *Combat Exposure Scale (CES)*

The Combat Exposure Scale (CES) is a seven-item self-report measure that assesses wartime stressors experienced by combatants. Items are rated on a five-point frequency (1 "no" or "never" to 5 "more than 50 times"), five-point duration (1 "never" to 5 "more than 6 months"), four-point frequency (1 "no" to 4 "more than 12 times") or four-point degree of loss (1 "no one" to 4 "more than 50%") scale. Respondents are asked to respond based on their exposure to various combat situations, such as firing rounds at the enemy and being on dangerous duty. The total CES score (ranging from 0 to 41) is calculated by using a sum of weighted scores, which can be classified into one of five categories of combat exposure ranging from "light" to "heavy." The CES was developed to be easily administered and scored and is useful in both research and clinical settings.

SAMPLE ITEM

Were you ever surrounded by the enemy? (1 "no" to 5 "more than 12 times").

### *Life Events Checklist (LEC)*

The Life Events Checklist (LEC) is a brief, seventeen-item, self-report measure designed to screen for potentially traumatic events in a respondent's lifetime.

The LEC assesses exposure to sixteen events known to potentially result in PTSD or distress and includes one item assessing any other extraordinarily stressful event not captured in the first sixteen items. For each item, respondents check whether the event (a) happened to them personally, (b) they witnessed the event, (c) they learned about the event, (d) they are not sure if the item applies to them, and (e) the item does not apply to them.

The LEC was developed concurrently with the Clinician Administered PTSD Scale (CAPS) and is administered before the CAPS. The LEC has demonstrated adequate psychometric properties as a stand-alone assessment of traumatic exposure, particularly when evaluating consistency of events that actually happened to a respondent. The LEC has also demonstrated convergent validity with measures assessing varying levels of exposure to potentially traumatic events and psychopathology known to relate to traumatic exposure.

However, the LEC does not establish that the respondent has experienced an event with sufficient severity to meet DSM-IV criteria for a traumatic exposure (Criterion A1), and it does not assess peritraumatic emotional experiences (Criterion A2).

#### SCORING

Items in which the respondent endorsed that the event happened to him or her personally receive a score of 1; all other responses receive a score of 0. Item scores are summed for a total score.

#### EXAMPLE ITEM

"Natural disaster (for example, flood, hurricane, tornado, earthquake)."

### *What Is the Difference Between a Trauma-Exposure Measure and a PTSD Measure?*

The purpose of a trauma-exposure measure is to identify what traumatic events an individual has experienced; the purpose of a PTSD measure is to determine whether the person has PTSD symptoms related to one of the identified events. There are a variety of trauma-exposure measures. Some are very broad and assess a range of negative life events as well as traumatic experiences.

Others have a narrower focus and only assess Criterion A, traumas that involve life threat. Similarly, there are a range of PTSD measures that can be broad enough to include symptoms other than those related to PTSD.

There are also PTSD measures that are more focused on the seventeen PTSD symptoms needed to make a diagnosis. In most cases, a thorough PTSD assessment involves the use of both a broad measure and a more focused measure.

### *What Are the Main Differences among PTSD Measures?*

PTSD measures vary in a number of ways. There are some basic differences to consider in terms of the (1) time required to administer the measure, (2) complexity of the format, (3) reading level of the person to be assessed, and (4) cost of use. Format is an important difference among measures. Measure formats range from seventeen-item self-report measures with a single rating for each item, to structured interviews with detailed inquiries about each symptom and interviewer ratings regarding the validity of reports. Structured interviews also differ in (1) whether they have a single gate-keeping item, (2) the level of sophistication for assessing each PTSD symptom, and (3) how well the ratings reflect symptom severity and/or frequency. Although interview measures require more interviewer training and administration time, they result in a more comprehensive assessment of PTSD. The right measure for a particular purpose depends on your goal. If you want a quick screen, a self-report measure may be best. However, if you are conducting a PTSD treatment study, you may want a sensitive interview that assesses for frequency and severity of symptoms.

### *What Are the Main Differences among Trauma-Exposure Measures?*

Trauma-exposure measures differ a great deal in length, the range of trauma types assessed, and the degree of detailed inquiry about each traumatic event. Many simply assess exposure to high-magnitude stressors that could cause traumatic stress, and others have detailed questions to follow up endorsed events. For example, one measure may have detailed questions about certain elements of an interpersonal violence experience, and another measure may only require a "yes" or "no" to the question of whether the person was exposed to a particular type of interpersonal violence. Some measures have been better validated than other measures, and some differ as to whether they assess the nature, degree, and duration of emotional responses to the stressor.

### *What Is the Best Measure for Assessing PTSD Symptoms?*

Some important considerations in choosing a PTSD measure include the time required to administer the measure, the reading level of the population being sampled, whether the desire is to assess symptoms related to a single traumatic event or to assess symptoms related to multiple traumatic events (or to assess symptoms when the trauma history is unknown), the need for the assessment to correspond to DSM criteria for PTSD, the psychometric strengths and weaknesses of the measure, and the cost of using the measure.

In addition, it is important that the overall complexity and language of the measure be appropriate to the population being sampled.

### *How Do I Choose a Measure to Assess Trauma History?*

It is difficult to assess trauma history because researchers cannot firmly establish the validity of trauma-exposure measures. It is so difficult to determine whether trauma reports are accurate that the validity of even the best measures has not been very rigorously studied. That being said, it seems likely that trauma-exposure assessments will have some validity, and their clinical relevance makes them necessary.

In choosing a measure of trauma history or exposure, there is generally a trade-off between the specificity of the assessed traumatic events and the length of the assessments. Measures that query about the widest range of potentially traumatic events, and presumably yield the most accurate reports, will be the longest. Measures that are quick and easy will inquire very broadly about types of events and may "miss" idiosyncratic traumatic events. Thus, in choosing a trauma-exposure measure for research, investigators will typically need to weigh the need for a detailed trauma-exposure assessment against the time limitations for the administration. Another consideration is whether the researcher is more interested in data regarding exposure to potentially traumatic (or high-magnitude) stressors or regarding exposures that resulted in significant emotional responses. Only a few measures assess the nature, degree, and duration of emotional responses to the stressor.

### *How Can I Obtain Trauma Exposure and PTSD Assessment Measures?*

The American Psychological Association's ethical guidelines on psychological test instruments require advanced graduate-level training in the administration and interpretation of psychodiagnostic assessment instruments. Thus, measures cannot be distributed to people who do not hold at least a master's degree in a clinical discipline. Graduate students must have a professor request the measure for them and use the measure under the professor's supervision.

In the Assessment section of the National Center for PTSD's website, you can find additional information about many measures, including a contact name and address for obtaining the measure. If the measure was developed by the National Center for PTSD, you can submit a request form to obtain the assessment tool.

## *Psychological Symptoms*

### PTSD SYMPTOMS

For many veterans, a diagnostic label may not be needed and may not facilitate treatment. In some circumstances, applying such a label may be counterproductive and undesirable to the veteran. A brief measure of PTSD symptoms can, however, be useful to get an idea of current PTSD symptoms a veteran might be having and to monitor treatment progress. A wide variety of brief measures of PTSD symptoms are available, and information about these (including contact information to obtain measures) can be found at www.ncptsd.va.gov.

Additional information about measures of PTSD can be found in Briere (1997), Carlson (1997), and Wilson and Keane (1996).

The Posttraumatic Checklist—Civilian (PCL-C) and the Screen for Posttraumatic Stress Symptoms (SPTSS) are measures that do not key symptoms to a particular event since exposure to multiple events is common and it is not clear that people can assign symptoms to events with any accuracy or that symptoms are, in fact, uniquely associated with particular events. The PCL-C is recommended rather than the PCL-Military because it is important to assess veterans' responses to military and nonmilitary traumatic events when assessing for treatment purposes. The SPTSS may be useful with veterans who have less formal education because it has a very low reading level. It may also be useful for veterans who are reluctant to report distress because it inquires about the frequency of symptoms rather than the degree of distress they cause.

If assignment of a diagnostic label is required or desired, the CAPS (Weathers, Keane, and Davidson, 2001) can be used. Detailed information about this structured interview and how to obtain it are available at www.ncptsd.va.gov.

*Dissociation* Dissociative symptoms are very common in trauma survivors, and they may not be spontaneously reported. The Trauma-Related Dissociation Scale (Carlson and Waelde 2000) is a measure of dissociation.

*Depression* Depression is a very common comorbid condition in those with posttraumatic disorders. It may be secondary to PTSD or associated with aspects of traumatic events such as losses. The Beck Depression Inventory (BDI)–Short Form is a common brief measure of depression (Beck and Steer 2000).

This measure is also available for computerized administration via the Decentralized Hospital Computer Program (DHCP) at VA medical centers.

*Traumatic Brief* Screen for Complicated Grief is a brief measure of symptoms of traumatic grief.

*Alcohol Use* Substance use is a common problem for those with PTSD, particularly alcohol abuse and dependence. The AUDIT (Goldman, Brown, and Christiansen 2000) is a screen for alcohol use. (For more information on alcohol abuse, see chapter 9.)

*Anger* Anger is a frequent problem for trauma survivors and outbursts of anger is a symptom of PTSD. If a veteran reports problems with anger, detailed assessment of that area may be useful.

The State-Trait Anger Expression Inventory (STAX-I) is measure of anger and how it is expressed (Spielberger 1988). This measure may be useful to assess veterans, although it is important to note that it is not ideal to assess recent, posttrauma anger because its trait form assesses both pretrauma and posttrauma anger and its state form assesses feelings at the time of the assessment (which may not be representative of the entire posttrauma period).

*Guilt and Shame* Guilt and shame are frequently issues for trauma survivors who feel distressed over what they did or did not do at the time of trauma. Kubany et al. (1995) have developed a measure of guilt that may be useful to assess those with clinical issues in that domain.

## *Relevant History*

### EXPOSURE TO POTENTIALLY TRAUMATIC EVENTS

Because exposure to previous traumatic stressors may affect response to traumatic stressors experienced in the military, it is important to broadly assess exposure to traumatic stressors. The Trauma History Screen (Carlson 2002) is a brief assessment tool that can be used for that purpose. Selected scales within the Deployment Risk and Resilience Inventory (DRRI; King, King, and Vogt 2003) may be used as a vehicle to identify particular combat and other high magnitude and threatening experiences that were potentially traumatic. Because the level of nontraumatic stressors and the overall context in which exposure to traumatic stressors occurs may affect the response to high magnitude stressors, it is important to assess these elements.

Several scales from the DRRI (e.g., concerns about life and family disruptions, difficult living and working environment, war-zone social support) may prove useful to gain a broader profile of the deployment experience.

FOR WOMEN VETERANS

Because women who serve in the military may be exposed to a number of traumatic stressors that are not assessed in combat measures, specific assessment of military stressors is often helpful for women veterans. The Life Stressors Checklist (Wolfe and Kimerling 1997) was developed for this purpose.

### *Treatment Options for PTSD*

The main treatments for people with PTSD are counseling (known as "talk" therapy or psychotherapy), medications, or both. Although there are a number of treatment options for PTSD, and patient response to treatment varies, some treatments have been shown to have more benefit in general. CBT is one type of counseling. With CBT, a therapist helps the service member dealing with PTSD understand and change how thoughts and beliefs about the trauma, and about the world, cause stress and maintain current symptoms. Table 3.1 describes several types of CBT.

CBT has been shown to be successful in treating PTSD in a number of well-controlled studies. However, there are a handful of service members for whom certain interventions may be inappropriate or for whom other treatment problems (e.g., co-occurring conditions) may also need to be addressed.

Visit this fact sheet from the VA National Center for PTSD for more information on cautions regarding cognitive-behavioral interventions within the first month of trauma. In addition to CBT, eye-movement desensitization and reprocessing (EMDR) is another type of therapy for PTSD. EMDR uses a combination of talk therapy with specific eye movements. Evidence of its effectiveness is mixed. In general, it appears that the talk therapy component is helpful, but most evidence suggests that the eye-movement component does not add much, if any, benefit. As with other kinds of counseling, the general psychotherapy component of EMDR can help change the reactions to memories service members experience as a result of their trauma(s).

### *Other PTSD Treatment Options*

As a new generation of service members returns from deployment, the DoD is faced with the challenge of identifying the most effective methods of treatment to address PTSD. Prevalence estimates of PTSD symptoms based on self-report surveys among OEF/OIF warriors vary, but it has clearly been shown to be a significant problem, especially for those exposed to sustained ground combat.

**Table 3.1 The Benefits of Different Types of Counseling in Treating PTSD**

| *Type of CBT* | *Overview/Components* | *Goal* |
|---|---|---|
| Prolonged Exposure Therapy | • Imaginal exposure: Repeated and prolonged recounting of the traumatic experience<br>• In vivo exposure: Systematic confrontation of trauma-related situations that are feared and avoided, despite being safe | Increase emotional processing of the traumatic event so that memories or situations no longer result in:<br>• Anxious arousal to trauma<br>• Escape and avoidance behaviors |
| Cognitive Therapy | • Modify the relationships between thoughts and feelings<br>• Identify and challenge inaccurate or extreme negatives thoughts<br>• Develop alternative, more logical or helpful thoughts | • Help the individual recognize and adjust trauma-related thoughts<br>• Help the individual modify his or her appraisal of self and the world |
| Cognitive Processing Therapy | Includes elements of Cognitive Therapy and Prolonged Exposure Therapy, including:<br>• Identifying and challenging problematic thoughts and beliefs (as noted above)<br>• Particular attention is paid to "stuck points": feelings, beliefs, and thoughts that stem from the traumatic events or are hard to accept<br>• Writing and reading aloud a detailed account of the traumatic event | • Help the individual modify beliefs about safety, trust, power/control, esteem, and intimacy<br>• Help the individual identify and modify "stuck points" |
| Stress Inoculation Training | • Provide a variety of coping skills that are useful in managing anxiety, including muscle relaxation, breathing retraining, and role playing, as well as cognitive techniques, such as guided self-talk<br>• May also include graduated in vivo exposure | • Decrease avoidance and anxious responding related to the trauma-related memories, thoughts, and feelings |

There are several treatment options that health professionals and clinicians can use to effectively treat service members with PTSD. Since there are a number of factors to consider in treating PTSD (e.g., access to services, availability, safety, patient preferences, etc.), it is important to understand the different types of treatments available to service members.

## PREVENTION

As with all conditions, successful prevention of PTSD would be more desirable than even the most effective treatment. To the extent that traumatic experiences themselves may be avoided, PTSD may sometimes be prevented.

In the immediate aftermath of traumatic exposure, preventive interventions are available, including psychoeducation, brief counseling, and prophylactic medication. Although some of these are promising, none has yet been proven to prevent PTSD.

A number of early interventions have been utilized for the prevention of PTSD. The most promising of these are public-health or population-based interventions informed by the evidence supporting CBT for PTSD. Psychological first aid is one example of a promising early intervention. Similarly, a growing number of well-controlled studies have demonstrated the effectiveness of CBT and exposure-based treatments as early interventions. Interventions such as these may decrease the likelihood of persons developing PTSD after traumatic exposures; however, additional research is needed to demonstrate this with certainty. Critical Incident Stress Debriefing (CISD) has been shown to be ineffective for the prevention of PTSD following trauma exposure and is not recommended in the current VA/DoD clinical practice guideline.

## ADDITIONAL TYPES OF COUNSELING

In addition to the treatments described above, other types of counseling may be helpful in treating PTSD.

Through group therapy, service members can talk about their trauma or learn skills to manage symptoms of PTSD (depending on the focus of the group). Many groups are effective and popular among those who have had similar traumatic experiences. Group therapy can help those with PTSD by giving them a chance to share their stories with others, feel more comfortable talking about their own trauma, and by enabling them to connect with others who have experienced similar problems or feelings. Some types of CBT can also be provided in a group setting.

Both family and couples therapies are methods of counseling that include the service member's family members. A therapist helps all of those

## Study Suggests PTSD May Be a Medical, Not Psychological Condition

Chicago Medical Innovations (CMI) is a nonprofit organization exclusively for medical, educational, charitable, and scientific purposes to research and implement effective, ongoing treatments for PTSD and Hot Flashes (HF). CMI is committed to treating both of these conditions as biological symptoms.

Dr. Eugene Lipov is the Medical Director of CMI and has developed neurobiological explanations for the origins of PTSD and HF. This is in addition to providing effective treatments for both highly debilitating conditions. His research findings have been replicated at multiple institutions such as Mayo Clinic, Belgium, Walter Reed Army Medical Center, and others.

CMI sponsors effective treatments to improve the Quality of Life (QoL) of patients with PTSD and HF. Additionally, CMI assists in the publication of the efficacy of the approaches for the treatments of the above conditions.

Their PTSD treatment technique involves stellate ganglion block (SGB) injections. After years of research it has been concluded by Dr. Lipov that the stellate ganglion (a collection of nerves) are connected to the insular amygdala and other cortical regions—parts of the brain largely responsible for PTSD. Applying an anesthetic to the ganglion reverses the effects of PTSD.

A local anesthetic (used in epidurals, which are often applied during labor) is injected to the nerves in the neck. Approximately thirty minutes after the treatment, patients experience relief from PTSD.

The FDA has ruled that approval for this treatment is not needed since SGB is a conventional procedure and uses a conventional anesthetic. While most drugs have a 50 percent compliance rate, this procedure has 100 percent compliance. The approach has been validated by the Walter Reed Army Medical Center.

In some cases patients can be weaned off all their psychiatric medications post treatment.

Dr. Lipov is an instructor with the Chicago-based North American Spine Society (NASS) and plans on training pain physicians and developing centers nationally to provide SGB to warfighters with PTSD.

SGB has been used since 1925, so the limitations and complications are well understood. A German study applied forty-five thousand SGBs and resulted in no permanent complications among patients.

The effects vary. Some patients have needed only one block and remain asymptomatic; others have found the block effective for a few months, requiring a second treatment, which effects, on those monitored, have lasted for two years. Patients remain off all related medications.

involved communicate, maintain good relationships, and cope with challenging emotions.

PTSD can sometimes have a significant negative impact on relationships, making this mode of therapy particularly helpful in some cases.

## PHARMACOLOGICAL APPROACHES

Selective serotonin reuptake inhibitors (SSRIs) are a type of antidepressant medication. SSRIs include citalopram (Celexa), fluoxetine (Prozac), paroxetine (Paxil), fluvoxamine (Luvox), and sertraline (Zoloft). Many, if not most, patients with PTSD will achieve some symptom relief with an SSRI, although the evidence of effectiveness is less convincing in combat PTSD compared to PTSD due to other traumas. Additional medications have been used for specific symptoms with some success. See the VA/DoD PTSD Clinical Practice Guidelines (CPGs) at www.healthquality.va.gov/ for additional information.

Prazosin may be promising for trauma-related nightmares. In addition, short-term use of a medication for sleep can be helpful for those who have significant difficulty sleeping immediately after a traumatic event. Longer-term use of sedative/hypnotic medications, such as benzodiazepines, however, has not been shown to be of benefit, and there is some evidence that long-term use of benzodiazepines in PTSD may interfere with psychotherapy.

## COMPLEMENTARY AND ALTERNATIVE MEDICINE

Complementary and alternative medicine (CAM) approaches to the treatment of many medical and mental health diagnoses, including PTSD, are in use; the research base to support their effectiveness is improving, but not complete. Acupuncture, a component of traditional Chinese medicine, has been examined for PTSD in a limited number of small RCTs. Although early results are promising, replication of these results in larger studies is needed. Yoga Nidra, a relaxation and meditative form of yoga, has also been used as an adjunctive treatment for PTSD. Formal studies demonstrating its effectiveness for PTSD are currently being conducted, and further research is needed on Yoga Nidra for PTSD before its effectiveness can be commented on.

Herbal or dietary supplements have also been used for the treatment of PTSD. Although there have been some studies of their effectiveness, the results of these small RCTs provide insufficient evidence to draw firm conclusions about their effectiveness for PTSD.

In addition, the quality and purity of herbals and dietary supplements available in the United States varies widely, further complicating their use. Revisions of the VA/DoD CPGs are currently under way to include a comprehensive review of the evidence for all treatments, including CAM.

### *Guidelines and Resources*

PTSD 101, made available by the VA's National Center for PTSD, is a web-based educational resource that is designed for practitioners who provide services to military men and women and their families as they recover from combat stress or other traumatic events.

#### ADDITIONAL RESOURCES

Center for the Study of Traumatic Stress
PTSD 101
Traumatic Grief: Symptomatology and Treatment for the Iraq War Veteran
PTSD in Iraq War Veterans: Implications for Primary Care
Treatment of Medical Casualty Evacuees
Traumatic Brain Injury and PTSD
Psychological First Aid: Field Operations Guide—SAMHSA
Readiness to Change in PTSD Treatment (video)
RESPECT-Mil Primary Care Physician's Manual
NACBT-Cognitive-Behavioral Therapy
Deployment Health Clinical Center—Medications
International Society for Traumatic Stress Studies—Treatment Guidelines

### *Assessment and Treatment of Anger in Combat-Related PTSD*

Casey T. Taft, PhD and Barbara L. Niles, PhD

Veterans of OIF who suffer from symptoms of PTSD are likely to have difficulties with anger regulation given the centrality of anger in the human survival response.

Research among military veterans has consistently shown that those with PTSD are higher in anger, hostility, aggression, general violence, and relationship violence and abuse than those without the disorder (e.g., Jordan et al. [1992]). "Irritability and outbursts of anger" represent one of the diagnostic criteria for PTSD and can have a debilitating impact across several domains.

Anger dysregulation typically has a deleterious impact on the veteran's relationships with family members and other loved ones, and may significantly interfere with other social and occupational functioning. These interpersonal difficulties may have a profound negative effect on the veteran's social support network, which places him or her at risk for PTSD exacerbation, and possibly for cardiovascular disease and other health problems that have been associated with anger, hostility, and PTSD. Angry outbursts may also place the veteran at risk for legal problems and may lead to severe consequences for those who are exposed to these outbursts.

Although little theory or research explicates the role of PTSD with respect to anger, one important theory for anger problems among veterans with PTSD emphasizes the role of context-inappropriate activation of cognitive processes related to a "survival mode" of functioning (Chemtob et al. 1997).

This response includes heightened arousal, a hostile appraisal of events, loss of the ability to engage in self-monitoring or other inhibitory processes, and resulting behavior produced to respond to this perceived severe threat.

These processes lead the veteran to see threats in the civilian environment that do not objectively pose any significant danger, and he or she may respond in an aggressive manner to such threats. This "survival mode," while adaptive in combat situations, typically becomes maladaptive when the individual interacts with his or her environment in civilian life. Therefore, in therapy with this population, an important treatment target often involves the detection of cognitive biases with respect to environmental threats and the detection of disconfirming evidence. This sense of heightened threat may be particularly acute among individuals who served in OIF because the enemy was not always clearly defined and military personnel were forced to be vigilant to attack at all times.

## ASSESSMENT OF ANGER AND RELATED CONSTRUCTS

Anger, hostility, and aggression are typically assessed via self-report questionnaire measures of these constructs. Two of the most widely used measures are the Buss Durkee Hostility Inventory (BDHI; Buss and Durkee 1957) and the STAX-I (Spielberger 1988).

The BDHI is the most widely used measure of hostility. The measure consists of seventy-five true-false items, and eight subscales: Assault, Indirect Hostility, Verbal Hostility, Irritability, Negativism, Resentment, Suspicion, and Guilt. The measure has received criticism based on methodological grounds (e.g., low predictive validity, poor reliability), and was recently revised by Buss and Perry (1992). The new measure, called the Aggression Questionnaire, consists of twenty-nine items that are rated on a five-point Likert scale. An advantage of this measure is that it taps not only anger, but also the related constructs of hostility and aggression. Specifically, subscales include Anger, Hostility, Verbal Aggression, and Physical Aggression.

This new measure and its subscales have been found to exhibit good psychometric properties.

The STAX-I is a forty-four-item measure that consists of subscales tapping State Anger, Trait Anger, and Anger Expression. This measure has some benefits over other existing anger measures. First, it distinguishes state anger and trait anger, and further distinguishes between the experience of anger and the expression of anger. Subscales can also be derived to assess whether individuals tend to keep in their anger (Anger-In), or express their anger openly (Anger-Out), or whether individuals effectively control and reduce their feelings of anger (Anger Control). These distinctions may be particularly important with veterans returning from Iraq. As described in the sections that follow, these men and women are likely to have problems with holding anger in and/or acting outwardly aggressive, and may vacillate between these two extremes. Therefore, this fine-grained assessment of the individual's anger expression style may assist in treatment planning.

## CHALLENGES FOR ANGER INTERVENTIONS

Veterans with PTSD frequently report that anger is one of their most troublesome problems, and anger often prompts their treatment entry. However, evidence suggests that anger and violence are often the precipitants for early termination from treatment, and higher anger levels are associated with poorer outcomes in treatment for PTSD more generally. This section highlights a number of important challenges for intervention with PTSD-positive veterans who have anger regulation problems.

For many who have served in OIF, the thought of openly discussing their difficulties with anger and finding alternatives to threatening or intimidating responses to everyday frustrations may seem to have life-threatening implications. The individual's anger and aggressive behavior may have been very functional in the military and in combat situations and may serve as a valuable source of self-esteem. Therefore, attempts to change an anger response may be met with considerable resistance. The advantages of disadvantages of the individual's anger-expression style should be discussed in order to move him or her in the direction of behavior change.

Generally, veterans will list several serious negative consequences of their anger regulation problems and few benefits that cannot be achieved by other, more appropriate means. Therefore, discussion of the "pros" and "cons" of their anger style often serves as a powerful technique for enhancing motivation.

Veterans may resist attempts to participate in treatment for anger problems because they may associate authority figures with distrust. Angry veterans may also become impatient during the treatment process due to their desire to gain relief from their anger problems and their general heightened level of hostility and frustration. They may become easily frustrated when changes do not immediately occur as a result of therapy, and may become hostile or otherwise resistant to therapy. It is important that the treatment provider fully discusses each of these concerns with the veteran, who should be encouraged to appropriately communicate his or her concerns during the course of treatment. Given the difficulty of the therapeutic endeavor, it is critical that the provider and veteran establish and maintain a positive therapeutic relationship. The provider should also be very clear in his or her expectations for treatment. He or she should stress to the veteran that one's anger expression style is learned, and the skills required to alter anger patterns will take time to master.

Several psychiatric problems tend to be highly comorbid with PTSD, such as depression and substance abuse. These problems also pose potential barriers for effective treatment of anger problems among those with PTSD. In addition, veterans with PTSD are more likely to suffer from physical health problems, and often suffer from severe social and occupational impairments.

These factors serve to increase stress and ameliorate emotional and tangible resources for the veteran, placing him or her at additional risk for anger dysregulation and violence perpetration. Furthermore, these factors may lead to a reduced ability to make use of treatment for anger problems. The veteran's capacity to marshal the cognitive resources to do the work of therapy (e.g., participate in self-monitoring exercises or practice communication skills) and to comply with the demands of treatment may be compromised. The treatment provider, therefore, must fully assess for comorbid problems and their impact on both the veteran's anger and his or her compliance with therapy, and should ensure that the veteran receives appropriate treatment for comorbid problems. For example, substance abuse must be addressed due to its disinhibiting effects with respect to anger and aggression.

## ANGER-MANAGEMENT INTERVENTION

Most PTSD treatment programs recommend and offer varied modalities and formats for the treatment of anger problems among veterans. Programs typically offer individual and group therapies, and cognitive-behavioral treatments for anger appear to be the most common.

Increasingly, PTSD programs are utilizing manualized or standardized group treatments for anger treatment, and there is some research evidence for the effectiveness of such treatments (Chemtob et al. 1997). Session content derived from a twelve-week standardized cognitive-behavioral group treatment for anger among veterans with PTSD is briefly outlined below.

Although this material derives from a group-treatment approach, the issues raised are relevant for other therapy formats and modalities.

*Overview of the Treatment* The goal of our anger-management group is for veterans to learn to understand and to better regulate their anger responses through greater awareness of their anger triggers and an application of constructive anger-management strategies. Additionally, veterans' appraisals of threat in their environment and daily experience of anger are targeted as they learn to prepare back-up responses (e.g., time-outs, relaxation, cognitive restructuring, ventilation, and positive distraction). Each session consists of group discussions and skills-building exercises. It has been found that each group of veterans presents with special needs and the sessions should be adapted accordingly. Group leaders vary their coverage of the material to best complement the unique needs of their group, and make efforts to encourage group cohesion and a safe and supportive group atmosphere.

The first two sessions of group discussion are devoted to orienting the veterans to treatment, discussing treatment goals and expectations of therapy, enhancing motivation to work on anger management, and providing psychoeducation on the anger response and the impact of PTSD on anger. Sessions 3 through 7 are devoted to self-monitoring exercises so that the veteran may better understand his or her anger response, developing an understanding of the distinction between different forms of anger expression, learning to use relaxation strategies for managing anger, and exploring motivational issues that may be impeding progress. The remaining sessions focus on communication skills and learning to communicate assertively, barriers to anger management posed by comorbid problems, and wrapping up.

*Setting Treatment Goals and Exploring Motivation* As discussed previously, it is extremely important that veterans with PTSD set realistic and attainable goals with respect to anger management, in order to prevent frustration with the therapy process and to reduce dropout. Both at the outset of therapy and throughout the course of treatment, motivational issues and barriers to successful barrier change should be explored. Also as discussed, for many veterans, anger dysregulation and aggressive behavior have served several adaptive functions, and anger expression styles may have been learned and reinforced throughout the life of the veteran.

Therefore, discussions should center not only on the negative consequences of anger dyscontrol, but also on those factors that are maintaining these maladaptive behaviors, as well as more adaptive behaviors that may serve as substitutes for identified problematic behaviors.

*Psychoeducation on Anger and PTSD* In order for veterans to better understand their anger dysregulation and to develop skills to better manage anger, it is important that they understand the constructs of anger and PTSD, and how the two are related. Veterans have often been noted to experience considerable relief upon the realization that their anger problems are directly related to their PTSD symptoms, and that others are experiencing the same difficulties. In addition to providing definitions of anger and PTSD, group leaders discuss the different components of the anger response (thoughts, emotions, physiology, and behaviors), and how these components are interrelated and negatively affected by PTSD.

Furthermore, it should be stressed that the goal of treatment is not to eliminate anger completely, since the anger response is a survival response that when communicated in a constructive manner, can be very useful and healthy.

Therefore, group leaders stress that the goal of anger treatment is to learn to manage anger better and express anger in an assertive manner.

*Self-monitoring* In order for veterans to learn new ways of handling their anger, they must first come to recognize when they are beginning to get angry, and recognize the thoughts and feelings associated with anger, as well as changes in their physiology. Many veterans returning from the war in Iraq may find this to be a difficult task, as their anger responses may be conditioned to respond immediately to the slightest risk of threat in their environment. That is, they may view their anger and aggression occurring instantly upon exposure to a perceived threat. However, upon completion of self-monitoring homework and in-group exercises, most group members learn to identify signs of anger (e.g., heart racing, thoughts of revenge, feelings of betrayal) prior to an angry outburst. It is very important for veterans to develop this recognition as early as possible in the anger cycle, so that they may take active steps to avoid escalation to aggression (e.g., by taking a time-out, using relaxation strategies, etc.). Self-monitoring exercises also provide important information regarding the veteran's perceptions of threat in his or her environment, which may be appropriately challenged in the therapy context.

*Assertiveness Training* Many veterans have learned to respond to threats or other potentially anger-provoking stimuli either in an aggressive manner (e.g., physical or verbal assaults) or in a passive manner. Veterans may fear their own aggressive impulses and may lack self-efficacy with respect to controlling their anger, and therefore, they are more likely to "stuff" their anger and avoid conflict altogether. Not surprisingly, this overly passive behavior often leads to feelings of resentment and a failure to resolve problems, which in turn, leads to a higher likelihood of subsequent aggressive behavior. Therefore, considerable time in treatment is devoted to making the distinctions clear between passive, aggressive, and assertive behavior, and group members are encouraged to generate and practice assertive responses to a variety of situations.

*Stress Management* In combating anger regulation problems, stress-management interventions are critical to reduce the heightened physiological arousal, anxiety, depression, and other comorbid problems that accompany PTSD and contribute to anger problems. In one protocol, an anger-arousal exercise is implemented, followed by a breathing-focused relaxation exercise to assist the veteran in becoming more aware of how thoughts are related to anger arousal and how relaxation exercises can assist in defusing the anger response.

The aim is to assist the veteran in creating an early warning system that will help him or her recognize and cope with anger before it escalates to aggressive behavior. In addition to the implementation of relaxation strategies, several other stress-management strategies are discussed and emphasized (e.g., self-care strategies, cognitive strategies) and the importance of social support in managing anger (e.g., talking with a friend or family member when angry) is stressed throughout the course of treatment.

*Communication-Skills Training* Anger dysregulation often results from a failure to communicate effectively and assertively, and likewise, heightened anger and PTSD hinder communication.

In our group treatment for anger problems, we cover several communication strategies (e.g., active listening, the "sandwich technique") and tips (e.g., using "I statements," paraphrasing, refraining from blaming or using threatening language) for effective communication. In this regard, it is important to emphasize both verbal and nonverbal communication, as veterans with PTSD often unknowingly use threatening or intimidating looks or gestures to maintain a safe distance from others.

### *Psychiatric Care in the Military Treatment System*

After first being air evacuated (AE) from the theater of war to Landstuhl Regional Medical Center in Germany, most patients may be sent to one of four stateside medical center regions. These include the Walter Reed National Military Medical Center (WRNMMC), Bethesda, Maryland; Dwight D. Eisenhower Army Medical Center, Fort Gordon, Georgia; Madigan Army Medical Center, Fort Lewis, Washington; and Brooke Army Medical Center, Fort Sam, Houston, Texas.

With some exceptions, this process is the same for Army, Navy, and Air Force personnel being air evacuated from the war zone. Patients who are AE but only require routine outpatient care are sent to the medical center closest to the site from which they were initially mobilized.

On arrival at the medical center, patients are triaged to ensure that outpatient care is, in fact, appropriate. They are then processed through the region's DHCC for further medical screening, and referred for treatment near their mobilization sites. While at the demobilization site, they continue to receive treatment and are evaluated for appropriate disposition. Veterans who require more intensive services are assigned to the medical center's Medical Holding Company and treated there.

Veterans who do not meet medical fitness standards are referred to a MEB. Those who are determined unsuitable either because of a preexisting condition or personality disorder are administratively separated. Those who are fit for duty with minor limitations are retained at the demobilization site for the remainder of their current term of service (reserve component) or released to their home duty station (active component).

A veteran requiring routine outpatient care usually remains at each echelon level hospital for seven to ten days until reaching his or her final destination.

Due to time constraints, treatment is generally focused on acute symptom relief and supportive therapy. Case management serves to identify appropriate resources to provide definitive treatments, when required.

Treatment availability varies from one site to the next. If a treatment modality is required and it is not offered at the final destination, consideration is given to the potential benefit of keeping a patient at the medical center for a longer period. More often than not, the military patient wishes to return home and does not want to delay the process any more than is necessary. In these cases, psychoeducation focuses on the early identification of symptoms and the importance of self-referral for rapid mental health intervention.

Any military patients requiring a MEB or who may require intensive outpatient care or inpatient care are air evacuated to a medical center. While programs vary with respect to available services, the process at WRNMMC serves as an example of treatment practices at the medical center level. WRNMMC offers several levels of mental health treatment. Upon arrival the on-call psychiatrist screens all air evacuated patients for acute symptoms that might necessitate hospitalization. Any patient air evacuated as an inpatient is admitted to the hospital and is continued in inpatient care until clinical safety is determined. During the course of the inpatient admission a comprehensive assessment is performed and treatment initiated.

Army personnel requiring an MEB remain at Walter Reed and are assigned to the Medical Holding Company. Air Force and Navy personnel undergoing an MEB may be followed in the WRNMMC Continuity Service within the partial hospitalization program until stabilized and ready for further disposition. Navy personnel undergoing an MEB are usually assigned to a medical holding unit near their home of record. Air Force personnel undergoing an MEB typically are returned to their unit. Inpatients with more severe illnesses and who are refractory to treatment may be discharged directly from the service to a VA inpatient ward near their home.

Outpatient follow-up is variable at all locations. Most if not all locations will have some form of treatment available. The WRNMMC mental health services are presented as a model of the process most mental health patients may experience in one form or another.

The WRNMMC Continuity Service offers several levels of care to include intensive outpatient services (defined as patients who require more than once-weekly therapy) and partial hospitalization (defined as daily treatment of at least three hours each day). Partial hospitalization serves as a step-down unit for inpatients transitioning to outpatient care or a step-up unit for outpatients who need more care than can be given in a routine outpatient setting.

Treatment modalities include group, individual, medication management, family and couples therapies as well as command consultations. Services are geared toward the needs of the patient. Daily war zone stress-related groups and individual therapies are available. Continuity Service also provides ongoing mental health treatment and case management for patients assigned to the Medical Holding Company to ensure effective psychiatric monitoring through the MEB process.

All Army mental health outpatients, whether they arrive as outpatients or are subsequently discharged from the inpatient service, are case managed by the Continuity Service until they leave WRNMMC. This ensures continuity of care and provides a resource that the patient can use during the time spent at WRNMMC. Those identified as primary mental health patients are monitored by the Continuity Service even if they are getting treatment on a different clinical service at WRNMMC.

The Behavioral Health Service is an outpatient treatment resource for "routine" ambulatory care, acute assessments, and liaison with military patients' units in the region. Treatments offered include individual and group therapies and medication management. Patient referrals come from the air-evacuation system, local units, and other medical specialties. The patient completes a comprehensive workup and an appropriate treatment plan is generated. Like the Inpatient and Continuity Service this can include return to duty, administrative separations, or referral to an MEB. Psychiatry Consultation and Liaison Service (PCLS) screens all hospitalized wounded in action (WIA) service members and most nonbattle injury (NBI) members. Disease nonbattle injury (DNBI) patients are also regularly evaluated by PCLS when requested through routine consultation. A mental health screening is performed on every patient admitted from the war zone and consists of a diagnostic interview and psychoeducation about combat stress, ASD, and PTSD.

Service members needing further psychiatric care are referred for treatment with PCLS, Continuity Services, or Behavioral Health as needed. Patients requiring administrative separation or an MEB may be delayed in separation from the service for several months. The types of treatments available throughout the DoD vary depending upon location and available resources. The patients may receive therapy from any of the modalities discussed above and may be involved in various treatment modalities while awaiting their final separation.

## DEMOBILIZATION—POSTDEPLOYMENT SCREENING

When service members return from deployment, regardless of whether due to normal troop rotation, medical evacuation, or for administrative reasons, they receive a comprehensive screening evaluation for presence of medical and psychiatric illness. This DoD-mandated Postdeployment Health Assessment (DD Form 2796) is performed either at the demobilization (DEMOB) site, or if a patient has been medically evacuated, at the Military Medical Center. This screening includes questions about depression, PTSD, and substance abuse. Individuals who screen positive are referred within seventy-two hours for a definitive mental health evaluation.

Service members with identified disorders are offered treatment and are evaluated for appropriate disposition. In the absence of nonpsychiatric conditions, aggressive treatment continues with the goal of retaining the individual and returning him or her to full duty. Service members are given an adequate trial of treatment before a decision is made to refer to the disability system through an MEB unless other conditions mandate referral to MEB.

## MEDICAL EVALUATION BOARD

If a service member requires evacuation from the combat zone for combat stress symptoms, the psychiatrist must decide whether the symptoms are due to a psychiatric condition, situational problem, or personality disorder. The psychiatrist must also determine the prognosis and likelihood of response to treatment. Generally, in the absence of a personality disorder or other confounding variables, aggressive treatment of combat stress reactions is indicated.

If the symptoms cannot be stabilized within a reasonable amount of time, then referral to a MEB is indicated for disability retirement. In deciding whether and when to initiate a MEB, the treating psychiatrist must consider the military patient's length of service, previous history, current symptoms, prognosis, as well as the time remaining on active duty for activated reservists. Junior ranking military members in their first enlistment with no prior deployment experience are likely to be referred to MEB. More seasoned military members are more likely to be monitored for up to one year with some duty limitations in an effort to retain them. Reservists who are nearing the end of their term of activation are likely to be allowed to be released from active duty (REFRAD) and referred for continued care and monitoring.

A service member may require referral to a MEB by virtue of his or her other medical conditions. When this is the case, a psychiatric addendum is performed to establish a service-connected condition, and to identify if the condition meets or does not meet medical retention standards.

One has to remain cognizant of the individual who may be attempting to manipulate the disability system in his or her favor by exaggerating symptoms, or seeking disability for conditions that are not medically unfitting.

The psychiatrist must be mindful of all motivating factors and the potential for the influence of a disability seeking culture.

## LIMITS OF MEDICAL AUTHORITY

It is important to be aware of the limitations physicians have when treating the military patient. The military physician's role is to treat the patient, determine if the patient is medically fit to fight, and make recommendations to the patient's commander about appropriate disposition. The only area where the physician has full authority is when a condition is life threatening, requires hospitalization, or does not meet retention standards and referral to MEB is indicated. In all other situations, the physician is a consultant to the system and can make recommendations only. Recommendations may include return to duty (RTD) without any limitations, RTD with some limitations or changes in environment, or administrative recommendations about rehabilitative or compassionate transfers, or discharge from the service.

Commanders have ultimate authority and bear ultimate responsibility for acting on recommendations. They may decide to attempt to rehabilitate a service member in his or her command despite recommendations for administrative discharge. A commander who chooses to ignore medical recommendations must review this decision with his or her higher commander. If the restrictions placed on a military member cannot be accommodated either by the nature of the mission or the individual's military occupational specialty (MOS), the commander may request a "Fitness for Duty Board" from the supporting hospital. If the service member is found fit with some limitations that constrain his or her duty performance, the commander may request evaluation by an MOS Medical Retention Board

(MMRB). The MMRB can return the warrior to duty, change the soldier's MOS, or refer him or her to the disability system.

## ETHICS OF MILITARY PSYCHIATRY

Military mental health officers must struggle with the ethical issues and duties to the individual and the military. They should always be the "honest broker" in caring for military patients and making tough decisions about treatment, referral to the disability system, administrative discharges, and limitations to duty. They must balance the mission requirements with the best interest of the patient and attempt to make the recommendation that will afford the service member the best outcome and opportunity for retention. Additionally, military mental health providers have got to recognize when the demands of service cannot afford the luxury of a prolonged rehabilitative period. They are also obligated to serve the interests of the service by remaining alert to secondary gain and malingering.

Military clinicians must understand that combat is one of life's most significant traumatic events.

They have to allow some vulnerable individuals to deploy and must recognize that some will become symptomatic. Ultimately, military mental health providers are required to remain empathic to the military patient as well as the needs of the service by providing compassionate treatment for combat veterans and referring service members who cannot be rehabilitated quickly to the disability system.

Clinicians involved in the treatment of casualties returning from OIF require an understanding of the military system in which these service members work and receive their medical care. Unlike prior conflicts, casualties from this war will likely receive treatment services in a variety of settings by providers from nonmilitary professional backgrounds.

Diversity within the military populations suggests that evacuated military patients are likely to come from different areas of the country and vary in terms of ethnic and cultural heritage. There is an increasing number of women as well. Patients' military experience may vary considerably depending upon the military component (e.g., active, reserve, or National Guard) to which these service members are assigned. They may have been exposed to a variety of different combat stressors, depending upon their site of duty, the nature of conflict to which they have been exposed, and the roles in which they have served. The literature is clear that certain psychiatric conditions, including ASDs and PTSD, are not uncommon responses to individuals exposed to combat. Clinicians must be aware of other psychiatric and organic disorders that might also contribute to their presentation, however.

The military system is designed to minimize psychiatric disorders on the battlefield through predeployment screening and by providing mental health services in the combat setting. When evacuation is required, service members may be treated within several echelons of care that are established.

Additionally, military regulation guides the appropriate evaluation of psychiatrically ill military patients. Service members with behavioral or emotional disorders may require discharge from service through the MEB process or through command determined administrative separation.

All of these factors can contribute to the clinical condition of an evacuated soldier, airman, or sailor. An appreciation of these complex issues will serve the clinician well in evaluating and treating service members psychiatrically evacuated from theater.

### *Treatment of the Returning War Veteran*

Josef I. Ruzek, PhD, Erika Curran, MSW, Matthew J. Friedman, MD, PhD, Fred D. Gusman, MSW, Steven M. Southwick, MD, Pamela Swales, PhD, Robyn D. Walser, PhD, Patrician J. Watson, PhD, and Julia Whealin, PhD.

It is important that VA and Vet Center clinicians recognize that the skills and experience that they have developed in working with veterans with chronic PTSD will serve them well with those returning from war. Their experience in talking about trauma, educating patients and families about traumatic stress reactions, teaching skills of anxiety and anger management, facilitating mutual support among groups of veterans, and working with trauma-related guilt will all be useful and applicable. The following section of this chapter highlights some challenges for clinicians, discusses ways in which care of these veterans may differ from the usual contexts of care, and directs attention to particular methods and materials that may be relevant to the care of the veteran recently traumatized in war.

#### THE HELPING CONTEXT: ACTIVE DUTY VS. VETERANS SEEKING HEATLH CARE

There are a variety of differences between the contexts of care for active duty military personnel and veterans normally being served in VA that may affect the way practitioners go about their business. First, many Iraq War patients will not be seeking mental health treatment. Some will have been evacuated for mental health or medical reasons and brought to VA, perhaps reluctant to acknowledge their emotional distress and almost certainly reluctant to consider themselves as having a mental health disorder (e.g., PTSD).

Second, emphasis on diagnosis as an organizing principle of mental health care is common in VA. Patients are given DSM-IV diagnoses, and diagnoses drive treatment. This approach may be contrasted with that of frontline psychiatry, in which pathologization of combat stress reactions is strenuously avoided. The strong assumption is that most will recover, and that their responses represent a severe reaction to the traumatic stress of war rather than a mental illness or disorder. According to this thinking, the "labeling" process may be counterproductive in the context of early care for Iraq War veterans.

As Koshes (1996) noted, "labeling a person with an illness can reinforce the 'sick' role and delay or prevent the soldier's return to the unit or to a useful role in military or civilian life" (p. 401).

Patients themselves may have a number of incentives to minimize their distress: to hasten discharge, to accelerate a return to the family, to avoid compromising their military career or retirement. Fears about possible impact on career prospects are based in reality; indeed, some will be judged medically unfit to return to duty. Veterans may be concerned that a diagnosis of PTSD, or even ASD, in their medical record may harm their chances of future promotion, lead to a decision to not be retained, or affect type of discharge received. Some may think that the information obtained if they receive mental health treatment will be shared with their unit commanders, as is sometimes the case in the military.

To avoid legitimate concerns about possible pathologization of common traumatic stress reactions, clinicians may wish to consider avoiding, where possible, the assignment of diagnostic labels such as ASD or PTSD, and instead focus on assessing and documenting symptoms and behaviors. Diagnoses of acute or adjustment disorders may apply if symptoms warrant labeling.

Concerns about confidentiality must be acknowledged and steps taken to create the conditions in which patients will feel able to talk openly about their experiences, which may include difficulties with commanders, misgivings about military operations or policies, or possible moral concerns about having participated in the war. It will be helpful for clinicians to know who will be privy to information obtained in an assessment. The role of the assessment and who will have access to what information should be discussed with concerned patients.

Active duty service members may have the option to remain on active duty or to return to the war zone. Some evidence suggests that returning to work with one's cohort group during wartime can facilitate improvement of symptoms. Although their wishes may or may not be granted, service members often have strong feelings about wanting or not wanting to return to war. For recently activated National Guard and Reservists, issues may be somewhat different (Dunning 1996). Many in this population never planned to go to war and so may be faced with obstacles to picking up the life they "left." Whether active duty, National Guard, or Reservist, listening to and acknowledging their concerns will help empower them and inform treatment planning.

War patients entering residential mental health care will have come to VA through a process different from that experienced by "traditional" patients. If they have been evacuated from the war zone, they will have been rapidly moved through several levels of medical triage and treatment, and treated by a variety of health care providers (Scurfield and Tice 1991). Many will have received some mental health care in the war zone (e.g., stress debriefing) that will have been judged unsuccessful. Some veterans will perceive their need for continuing care as a sign of personal failure. Understanding their path to VA will help the building of a relationship and the design of care.

More generally, the returning soldier is in a state of transition from war zone to home, and clinicians must seek to understand the expectations and consequences of returning home for the veteran. Is the veteran returning to an established place in society, to an economically deprived community, to a supportive spouse or cohesive military unit, to a large impersonal city, to unemployment, to financial stress, to an American public thankful for his or her sacrifice?

Whatever the circumstances, things are unlikely to be as they were: "The deployment of the family member creates a painful void within the family system that is eventually filled (or denied) so that life can go on. . . . The family assumes that their experiences at home and the soldier's activities on the battlefield will be easily assimilated by each other at the time of reunion and that the pre-war roles will be resumed. The fact that new roles and responsibilities may not be given up quickly upon homecoming is not anticipated" (Yerkes and Holloway 1996, 31).

## LEARNING FROM VIETNAM VETERANS WITH CHRONIC PTSD

From the perspective of work with Vietnam veterans whose lives have been greatly disrupted by their disorder, the chance to work with combat veterans soon after their war experiences represents a real opportunity to prevent the development of a disastrous life course. We have the opportunity to directly focus on traumatic stress reactions and PTSD symptom reduction (e.g., by helping veterans process their traumatic experiences, by prescribing medications) and thereby reduce the degree to which PTSD, depression, alcohol/substance misuse, or other psychological problems interfere with quality of life. We also have the opportunity to intervene directly in key areas of life functioning, to reduce the harm associated with continuing posttraumatic stress symptoms and depression if those prove resistant to treatment.

The latter may possibly be accomplished via interventions focused on actively supporting family functioning in order to minimize family problems, reducing social alienation and isolation, supporting workplace functioning, and preventing use of alcohol and drugs as self-medication (a different focus than addressing chronic alcohol or drug problems).

### PREVENT FAMILY BREAKDOWN

At time of return to civilian life, they can face a variety of challenges in reentering their families, and the contrast between the fantasies and realities of homecoming (Yerkes and Holloway 1996) can be distressing. Families themselves have been stressed and experienced problems as a result of the deployment (Norwood, Fullerton, and Hagen 1996).

Partners have made role adjustments while the soldier was away, and these need to be renegotiated, especially given the possible irritability and tension of the veteran (Kirkland 1995). The possibility exists that mental health providers can reduce long-term family problems by helping veterans and their families anticipate and prepare for family challenges, involving families in treatment, providing skills training for patients (and where possible, their families) in family-relevant skills (e.g., communication, anger management, conflict resolution, parenting), providing short-term support for family members, and linking families together for mutual support.

### PREVENT SOCIAL WITHDRAWAL AND ISOLATION

PTSD also interferes with social functioning. Here the challenge is to help the veteran avoid withdrawal from others by supporting reentry into existing relationships with friends, work colleagues, and relatives, or where appropriate, assisting in development of new social relationships. The latter may be especially relevant with individuals who leave military service and transition back into civilian life. Social functioning should be routinely discussed with patients and made a target for intervention. Skills training focusing on the concrete management of specific difficult social situations may be very helpful. Also, as indicated below, clinicians should try to connect veterans with other veterans in order to facilitate the development of social networks.

### PREVENT PROBLEMS WITH EMPLOYMENT

Associated with chronic combat-related PTSD have been high rates of job turnover and general difficulty in maintaining employment, often attributed by veterans themselves to anger and irritability, difficulties with authority, PTSD symptoms, and substance abuse. Steady employment, however, is likely to be one predictor of better long-term functioning, as it can reduce financial stresses, provide a source of meaningful activity and self-esteem, and give opportunities for companionship and friendship. In some cases, clinicians can provide valuable help by supporting the military or civilian work functioning of veterans, by teaching skills of maintaining or, in the case of those leaving the military, finding of employment, or facilitating job-related support groups.

### PREVENT ALCOHOL AND DRUG ABUSE

The comorbidity of PTSD with alcohol and drug problems in veterans is well established (Ruzek 2003). Substance abuse adds to the problems caused by PTSD and interferes with key roles and relationships, impairs coping, and impairs entry into and ongoing participation in treatment. PTSD providers are aware of the need to routinely screen and assess for alcohol and drug use, and are knowledgeable about alcohol and drug (especially 12-Step) treatment.

Many are learning, as well, about the potential usefulness of integrated PTSD-substance-abuse treatment, and the availability of manualized treatments for this dual disorder. Seeking Safety, a structured group protocol for trauma-relevant coping skills training (Najavits 2002), is seeing increased use in VA and should be considered as a treatment option for Iraq War veterans who have substance use disorders along with problematic traumatic-stress responses. In addition, for many newly returning Iraq War veterans, it will be important to supplement traditional abstinence-oriented treatments with attention to milder alcohol problems, and in particular to initiate preventive interventions to reduce drinking or prevent acceleration of alcohol consumption as a response to PTSD symptoms (Bien, Miller, and Tonigan 1993). For *all* returning veterans, it will be useful to provide education about safe drinking practices and the relationship between traumatic stress reactions and substance abuse.

### GENERAL CONSIDERATIONS IN CARE

*Connect with the Returning Veteran* As with all mental health counseling, the relationship between veteran and helper will be the starting point for care. Forming a working alliance with some returnees may be challenging, however, because most newly returned veterans may be, as Litz (2002) notes, "defended, formal, respectful, laconic, and cautious" and reluctant to work with the mental health professional. Especially in the context of recent exposure to war, validation (Kirkland 1995) of the veteran's experiences and concerns will be crucial. Discussion of "war zone," not "combat," stress may be warranted because some traumatic stressors (e.g., body handling, sexual assault) may not involve war fighting as such. Thought needs to be given to making the male-centric hospital system hospitable for women, especially for women who have experienced sexual assault in the war zone, for whom simply walking onto the grounds of a VA hospital with the ubiquitous presence of men may create feelings of vulnerability and anxiety.

Practitioners should work from a patient-centered perspective, and take care to find out the current concerns of the patient (e.g., fear of returning to the war zone, concerns about having been evacuated and what this means, worries about reactions of unit, fear of career ramifications, concern about reactions of family, concerns about returning to active duty). One advantage of such an orientation is that it will assist with the development of a helping relationship.

*Connect Veterans with Each Other* In treatment of chronic PTSD, veterans often report that perhaps their most valued experience was the opportunity to connect in friendship and support with other vets. This is unlikely to be different for returning Iraq War veterans, who may benefit greatly from connection both with each other and with veterans of other conflicts. Fortunately, this is a strength of VA and Vet Center clinicians, who routinely and skillfully bring veterans together.

*Offer Practical Help with Specific Problems* Returning veterans are likely to feel overwhelmed with problems related to workplace, family and friends, finances, physical health, and so on. These problems will be drawing much of their attention away from the tasks of therapy, and may create a climate of continuing stress that interferes with resolution of symptoms. The presence of continuing negative consequences of war deployment may help maintain posttraumatic stress reactions.

Rather than treating these issues as distractions from the task at hand, clinicians can provide a valuable service by helping veterans identify, prioritize, and execute action steps to address their specific problems.

*Attend to Broad Needs of the Person* Wolfe, Keane, and Young (1996) put forward several suggestions for clinicians serving Persian Gulf War veterans that are also important in the context of the Iraq War. They recommended attention to the broad range of traumatic experience. They similarly recommended broad clinical attention to the impact of both premilitary and postmilitary stressors on adjustment.

For example, history of trauma places those exposed to trauma in the war zone at risk for development of PTSD, and in some cases war experiences will activate emotions experienced during earlier events. Finally, recognition and referral for assessment of the broad range of physical health concerns and complaints that may be reported by returning veterans is important.

Mental health providers must remember that increased health symptom reporting is unlikely to be exclusively psychogenic in origin (Proctor et al. 1998).

## METHODS OF CARE: OVERVIEW

Management of acute stress reactions and problems faced by recently returned veterans are highlighted below. Methods of care for the Iraq War veteran with PTSD are similar to those provided to veterans with chronic PTSD.

## EDUCATION ABOUT POSTTRAUMATIC STRESS REACTIONS

Education is a key component of care for the veteran returning from war experience and is intended to improve understanding and recognition of symptoms, reduce fear and shame about symptoms, and, generally, "normalize" his or her experience. It should also provide the veteran with a clear understanding of how recovery is thought to take place, what will happen in treatment, and, as appropriate, the role of medication.

With such understanding, stress reactions may seem more predictable and fears about long-term effects can be reduced. Education in the context of relatively recent traumatization (weeks or months) should include the conception that many symptoms are the result of psychobiological reactions to extreme stress and that, with time, these reactions, in most cases, will diminish.

Reactions should be interpreted as responses to overwhelming stress rather than as personal weakness or inadequacy. In fact, some recent research (e.g., Steil and Ehlers 2000) suggests that survivors' own responses to their stress symptoms will in part determine the degree of distress associated with those symptoms and whether they will remit. Whether, for example, posttrauma intrusions cause distress may depend in part on their meaning for the person (e.g., "I'm going crazy").

## TRAINING IN COPING SKILLS

Returning veterans experiencing recurrent intrusive thoughts and images, anxiety and panic in response to trauma cues, and feelings of guilt or intense anger are likely to feel relatively powerless to control their emotions and thoughts. This helpless feeling is in itself a trauma reminder. Because loss of control is so central to trauma and its attendant emotions, interventions that restore self-efficacy are especially useful.

Coping-skills training is a core element in the repertoire of many VA and Vet Center mental health providers. Some skills that may be effective in treating Iraq War veterans include anxiety management (breathing retraining and relaxation), emotional "grounding," anger management, and communication.

However, the days, weeks, and months following the return home may pose specific situational challenges; therefore, a careful assessment of the veteran's current experience must guide selection of skills. For example, training in communication skills might focus on the problem experienced by a veteran in expressing positive feelings toward a partner (often associated with emotional numbing); anger management could help the veteran better respond to others in the immediate environment who do not support the war.

Whereas education helps survivors understand their experience and know what to do about it, coping skills training should focus on helping them know *how* to do the things that will support recovery. It relies on a cycle of instruction that includes education, demonstration, rehearsal with feedback and coaching, and repeated practice. It includes regular between-session task assignments with diary self-monitoring and real-world practice of skills. It is this repeated practice and real-world experience that begins to empower the veteran to better manage his or her challenges (see Najavits [2002] for a useful manual of trauma-related coping skills).

### EXPOSURE THERAPY

Exposure therapy is among the best-supported treatments for PTSD. It is designed to help veterans effectively confront their trauma-related emotions and painful memories, and can be distinguished from simple discussion of traumatic experience in that it emphasizes *repeated* verbalization of traumatic memories (see Foa and Rothbaum [1998] for a detailed exposition of the treatment). Patients are exposed to their own individualized fear stimuli repetitively, until fear responses are consistently diminished.

Often, in-session exposure is supplemented by therapist-assigned and monitored self-exposure to the memories or situations associated with traumatization.

In most treatment settings, exposure is delivered as part of a more comprehensive "package" treatment; it is usually combined with traumatic-stress education, coping-skills training, and, especially, cognitive restructuring (see below). Exposure therapy can help correct faulty perceptions of danger, improve perceived self-control of memories and accompanying negative emotions, and strengthen adaptive coping responses under conditions of distress.

### COGNITIVE RESTRUCTURING

Cognitive therapy or restructuring, one of the best-validated PTSD treatments (Foa et al. 2000), is designed to help the patient review and challenge distressing trauma-related beliefs. It focuses on educating participants about the relationships between thoughts and emotions, exploring common negative thoughts held by trauma survivors, identifying personal negative beliefs, developing alternative interpretations or judgments, and practicing new thinking. This is a systematic approach that goes well beyond simple discussion of beliefs to include individual assessment, self-monitoring of thoughts, homework assignments, and real-world practice. In particular, it may be a most helpful approach to a range of emotions other than fear—guilt, shame, anger, depression—that may trouble veterans. For example, anger may be fueled by negative beliefs (e.g., about perceived lack of preparation or training for war experiences, about harm done to their civilian career, about perceived lack of support from civilians). Cognitive therapy may also be helpful in helping veterans cope with distressing changed perceptions of personal identity that may be associated with participation in war or loss of wartime identity upon return (Yerkes and Holloway 1996).

A useful resource is the *Cognitive Processing Therapy* manual developed by Resick and Schnicke (1993), which incorporates extensive cognitive restructuring and limited exposure. Although designed for application to rape-related PTSD, the methods can be easily adapted for use with veterans. Kubany's (1998) work on trauma-related guilt may be helpful in addressing veterans' concerns about harming or causing death to civilians.

### FAMILY COUNSELING

Mental health professionals within VA and Vet Centers have a long tradition of working with family members of veterans with PTSD. This same work, including family education, weekend family workshops, couples counseling, family therapy, parenting classes, or training in conflict resolution, will be very important with Iraq War veterans.

### PHARMACOTHERAPY

*Pharmacologic Treatment of Acute Stress Reactions* Pharmacological treatment for acute stress reactions (within one month of the trauma) is generally reserved for individuals who remain symptomatic after having already received brief crisis-oriented psychotherapy. This approach is in line with the deliberate attempt by military professionals to avoid medicalizing stress-related symptoms and to adhere to a strategy of immediacy, proximity, and positive expectancy.

Prior to receiving medication for stress-related symptoms, the war zone survivor should have a thorough psychiatric and medical examination, with special emphasis on medical disorders that can manifest with psychiatric symptoms (e.g., subdural hematoma, hyperthyroidism), potential psychiatric disorders (e.g., ASD, depression, psychotic disorders, panic disorder), use of alcohol and substances of abuse, use of prescribed and over-the-counter medication, and possible drug allergies. It is important to assess the full range of potential psychiatric disorders, and not just PTSD, since many symptomatic service personnel will be at an age when first episodes of schizophrenia, mania, depression, and panic disorder are often seen.

In some cases a clinician may need to prescribe psychotropic medications even before completing the medical or psychiatric examination. The acute use of medications may be necessary when the patient is dangerous, extremely agitated, or psychotic. In such circumstances the patient should be taken to an emergency room; short-acting benzodiazepines (e.g., lorazepam) or high-potency neuroleptics (e.g., Haldol) with minimal sedative, anticholinergic, and orthostatic side effects may prove effective. Atypical neuroleptics (e.g., risperidone) may also be useful for treating aggression.

When a decision has been made to use medication for acute stress reactions, rational choices may include benzodiazepines, antiadrenergics, or antidepressants. Shortly after traumatic exposure, the brief prescription of benzodiazepines (four days or less) has been shown to reduce extreme arousal and anxiety and to improve sleep. However, early and prolonged use of benzodiazepines is contraindicated, since benzodiazepine use for two weeks or longer has actually been associated with a higher rate of subsequent PTSD.

Although antiadrenergic agents including clonidine, guanfacine, prazosin, and propranolol have been recommended (primarily through open nonplacebo controlled treatment trials) for the treatment of hyperarousal, irritable aggression, intrusive memories, nightmares, and insomnia in survivors with chronic PTSD, there is only suggestive preliminary evidence of their efficacy as an acute treatment. Of importance, antiadrenergic agents should be prescribed judiciously for trauma survivors with cardiovascular disease due to potential hypotensive effects and these agents should also be tapered, rather than discontinued abruptly, in order to avoid rebound hypertension.

Furthermore, because antiadrenergic agents might interfere with counter-regulatory hormone responses to hypoglycemia, they should not be prescribed to survivors with diabetes.

Finally, the use of antidepressants may make sense within four weeks of war, particularly when trauma-related depressive symptoms are prominent and debilitating. To date, there has been one published report on the use of antidepressants for the treatment of ASD. Recently traumatized children meeting criteria for ASD who were treated with imipramine for two weeks experienced significantly greater symptom reduction than children who were prescribed chloral hydrate.

*Pharmacologic Treatment of Posttraumatic Stress Disorder* Pharmacotherapy is rarely used as a stand-alone treatment for PTSD and is usually combined with psychological treatment. The following text briefly presents recommendations for the pharmacotherapeutic treatment of PTSD.

Findings from subsequent large-scale trials with paroxetine have demonstrated that SSRI treatment is clearly effective both for men in general and for combat veterans suffering with PTSD.

We recommend SSRIs as first-line medications for PTSD pharmacotherapy in men and women with military-related PTSD. SSRIs appear to be effective for all three PTSD symptom clusters in both men and women who have experienced a variety of severe traumas and they are also effective in treating a variety of comorbid psychiatric disorders, such as major depression and panic disorder, which are commonly seen in individuals suffering with PTSD. Additionally, the side effect profile with SSRIs is relatively benign (compared to most psychotropic medications) although arousal and insomnia may be experienced early on for some patients with PTSD.

Second-line medications include nefazadone, tricyclic antidepressants (TCAs), and monoamine oxidase inhibitors (MAOIs). Evidence favoring the use of these agents is not as compelling as for SSRIs because fewer subjects have been tested at this point. The best evidence from open trials supports the use of nefazadone, which like SSRIs promotes serotonergic actions and is less likely than SSRIs to cause insomnia or sexual dysfunction.

Trazadone, which has limited efficacy as a stand-alone treatment, has proven very useful as augmentation therapy with SSRIs; its sedating properties make it a useful bedtime medication that can antagonize SSRI-induced insomnia.

Despite some favorable evidence of the efficacy of MAOIs, these compounds have received little experimental attention since 1990.

Venlafaxine and bupropion cannot be recommended because they have not been tested systematically in clinical trials. There is a strong rationale from laboratory research to consider antiadrenergic agents. It is hoped that more extensive testing will establish their usefulness for PTSD patients. The best research on this class of agents has focused on prazosin, which has produced marked reduction in traumatic nightmares, improved sleep, and global improvement in veterans with PTSD. Hypotension and sedation need to be monitored. Patients should not be abruptly discontinued from antiadrenergics. Despite suggestive theoretical considerations and clinical findings, there is only a small amount of evidence to support the use of carbamazepine or valproate with PTSD patients. Furthermore, the complexities of clinical management with these effective anticonvulsants have shifted current attention to newer agents (e.g., gabapentin, lamotrigine, and topirimate), which have yet to be tested systematically with PTSD patients.

Benzodiazepines cannot be recommended for patients with PTSD. They do not appear to have efficacy against core PTSD patients. No studies have demonstrated efficacy for PTSD-specific symptoms.

Conventional antipsychotics cannot be recommended for PTSD patients. Preliminary results suggest, however, that atypical antipsychotics may be useful, especially to augment treatment with first- or second-line medications, especially for patients with intense hypervigilance or paranoia, agitation, dissociation, or brief psychotic reactions associated with their PTSD. As for side effects, all atypicals may produce weight gain and olanzapine treatment has been linked to the onset of Type II diabetes mellitus.

*General Guidelines* Pharmacotherapy should be initiated with SSRI agents. Patients who cannot tolerate SSRIs or who show no improvement might benefit from nefazadone, MAOIs, or TCAs.

For patients who exhibit a partial response to SSRIs, one should consider continuation or augmentation. A recent trial with sertraline showed that approximately half of all patients who failed to exhibit a successful clinical response after twelve weeks of sertraline treatment, did respond when SSRI treatment was extended for another twenty-four weeks. Practically speaking, clinicians and patients usually will be reluctant to stick with an ineffective medication for thirty-six weeks, as in this experiment. Therefore, augmentation strategies seem to make sense. Here are a few suggestions based on clinical experience and pharmacological "guesstimates," rather than on hard evidence:

- Excessively aroused, hyperreactive, or dissociating patients might be helped by augmentation with an antiadrenergic agent.
- Labile, impulsive, and/or aggressive patients might benefit from augmentation with an anticonvulsant.
- Fearful, hypervigilant, paranoid, and psychotic patients might benefit from an atypical antipsychotic.

## INTEGRATING INTO EXISTING SPECIALIZED PTSD SERVICES

War service members with stress-related problems may need to be integrated into existing VA PTSD Residential Rehabilitation Programs or other VA mental health programs. Approaches to this integration of psychiatric evacuees vary and each receiving site needs to determine its own "best fit" model for provision of services and integration of veterans. At the National Center's PTSD Residential Rehabilitation Program in the VA Palo Alto Health Care System, it is anticipated that Iraq War patients will generally be integrated with the rest of the milieu (e.g., for community meetings, affect-management classes, conflict resolution, communication-skills training), with the exception of identified treatment components. The latter elements of treatment, in which Iraq War veterans will work together, will include process, case management, and acute stress/PTSD education groups (and, if delivered in groups, exposure therapy, cognitive restructuring, and family/couples counseling). The thoughtful mixing of returning veterans with veterans from other wars/conflicts is likely, in general, to enhance the treatment experience of both groups.

### PRACTITIONER ISSUES

Working with Iraq War veterans affected by war zone trauma is likely to be emotionally difficult for therapists. It is likely to bring up many feelings and concerns—reactions to stories of death and great suffering, judgments about the morality of the war, reactions to patients who have killed, feelings of personal vulnerability, feelings of therapeutic inadequacy, perceptions of a lack of preparation for acute care—that may affect ability to listen empathically to the patient and maintain the therapeutic relationship (Sonnenberg 1996). Koshes (1996) suggested that those at greatest risk for strong personal reactions might be young, inexperienced staff who are close in age to patients and more likely to identify with them, and technicians or paraprofessional workers who may have less formal education about the challenges associated with treating these patients but who actually spend the most time with patients.

Regardless of degree of experience, all mental health workers must monitor themselves and practice active self-care, and managers must ensure that training, support, and supervision are part of the environment in which care is offered.

## *PTSD in War Veterans: Implications for Primary Care*

Annabel Prins, PhD, Rachel Kimerling, PhD, and Gregory Leskin, PhD

During and after the Iraq War, primary care providers may notice changes in their patient population. There may be an increased number of veterans or active duty military personnel returning from the war. There also may be increased contact with family members of active duty personnel, including family members who have lost a loved one in the war or family members of individuals missing in action or taken prisoner of war. In addition, there may be increased distress in veterans of other wars, conflicts, and peacekeeping missions. All of these patients may be experiencing symptoms of posttraumatic stress disorder (PTSD):

- Veterans and active duty military personnel may have witnessed or participated in frightening and upsetting aspects of combat.
- Veterans and active duty military personnel may have experienced military-related sexual trauma during their service.
- Family members may suffer traumatic stress by hearing about frightening or upsetting events that happened to loved ones, or from the loss or fears of loss related to family members missing or deceased.
- Other veterans may be reminded of frightening and upsetting experiences from past wars, which can exacerbate traumatic stress responses.

These types of stress reactions often lead people to increase their medical utilization. Because far fewer people experiencing traumatic-stress reactions seek mental health services, primary care providers are the health professionals with whom individuals with PTSD are most likely to come into contact.

### WHAT DO PRIMARY CARE PRACTITIONERS NEED TO KNOW ABOUT PTSD? PATIENTS WANT PRIMARY CARE PROVIDERS TO ACKNOWLEDGE THEIR TRAUMATIC EXPERIENCES AND RESPONSES

- Over 90 percent of patients indicate that traumatic experiences and responses are important and relevant to their primary care.
- Over 90 percent of patients in VA primary care settings will have experienced at least one traumatic event in their life. Most will have experienced four or more.
- The relationship between trauma exposure and increased health care utilization appears to be mediated by the diagnosis of PTSD.
- Thus, primary care practitioners should be aware of the essential features of PTSD: reexperiencing symptoms (e.g., nightmares, intrusive thoughts), avoidance of trauma cues, numbing/detachment from others, and hyperarousal (e.g., increased startle, hypervigilance).

### PTSD CAN BE DETECTED IN PRIMARY CARE SETTINGS

- The Primary Care PTSD (PC-PTSD) screen can be used to detect PTSD in primary care.
- Endorsement of any three items is associated with a diagnostic accuracy of .85 (sensitivity .78; specificity .87) and indicates the need for additional assessment.

## PTSD CAN BE EFFECTIVELY MANAGED IN PRIMARY CARE SETTINGS

By recognizing patients with PTSD and other trauma-related symptoms you can

- Provide patients and their family members with educational materials that help them understand that their feelings are connected to the Iraq War and its consequences.
- Validate patients' distress, and help them know that their feelings are not unusual in these circumstances.
- When appropriate, initiate treatment for PTSD or mental health consultation.

## WHAT CAN PRIMARY CARE PROVIDERS DO FOR THEIR PATIENTS?

*Determine the Patient's Status in Relationship to the War* By assessing the patient's status in relation to the war, primary care providers acknowledge the relevance and importance of this event. Example questions include

"Have you recently returned from the Persian Gulf? How has your adjustment been?"

"Do you have family members or friends who are currently in the Persian Gulf? How are you dealing with their absence?"

"How has the war in Iraq affected your functioning?"

*Acknowledge the Patient's Struggles* Regardless of their specific relationship to the war, primary care providers should recognize and normalize distress associated with war. Example statements include:

"I am so sorry that you are struggling with this."

"I can appreciate how difficult this is for you."

"You are not the only patient I have who is struggling with this."

"It's not easy, is it?"

*Assess for PTSD Symptoms* The PC-PTSD can be used either as a self-report measure or through interview. It can be a standard part of a patient information form or introduced as follows:

"I would like to know if you are experiencing any specific symptoms."

"It is not uncommon for people to have certain types of reactions. I would like to know if . . ."

*Be Aware of How Trauma May Impact on Medical Care* The specific health problems associated with PTSD are varied and suggest multiple etiologies; neurobiological, psychological, and behavioral factors are likely explanations. Research has increasingly demonstrated that PTSD can lead to neurobiological dysregulation, altering the functioning of catecholamine, hypothalamic-pituitary-adrenocorticoid, endogenous opioid, thyroid, immune, and neurotransmitter systems.

Exposure to traumatic stress is associated with increased health complaints, health-service utilization, morbidity, and mortality. PTSD appears to be a key mechanism that accounts for the association between trauma and poor health.

PTSD and exposure to traumatic experiences are associated with a variety of health-threatening behaviors, such as alcohol and drug use, risky sexual practices, and suicidal ideation and gestures.

PTSD is associated with an increased number of both lifetime and current physical symptoms, and PTSD severity is positively related to self-reports of physical conditions.

*Determine If and How Trauma Responses Can Be Managed in PC* The delivery of mental health care is possible in the general or primary care setting. According to this approach, brief psychotherapeutic, psychoeducational, and pharmacological services are delivered as a "first-line" intervention to primary care patients. If a patient fails to respond to this level of intervention, or obviously needs specialized treatment (e.g., presence of psychotic symptoms or severe dissociative symptoms), the patient is referred to mental health emergency, outpatient mental health intake coordinator, or PTSD program.

### PROCEDURES TO FOLLOW IF PATIENT DEMONSTRATES PTSD

*Symptoms during Medical Examination* Medical examinations or procedures may cause the patient to feel anxious or panicky. The following techniques may help in addressing trauma-related symptoms that arise in the medical setting:

- Speak in a calm, matter-of-fact voice.
- Reassure the patient that everything is okay.
- Remind the patient that he or she is in a safe place and his or her care and well-being are a top priority.
- Explain medical procedures and check with the patient (e.g., "Are you ok?").
- Ask (or remind) the patient where he or she is right now.
- If the patient is experiencing flashbacks, remind him or her that they are in a doctor's office at a specific time in a specific place (grounding).
- Offer the patient a drink of water, an extra gown, or a warm or cold washcloth for the face, anything that will make the patient feel more like his or her usual self.
- Any assistance and sensitivity on the part of the primary care provider can help reinforce an effective and positive alliance with the patient.

## ADDITIONAL RESOURCES

To learn more about screening and treatment for PTSD in primary care settings, additional educational materials are available at the following websites:

- Posttraumatic Stress Disorder: Implications for Primary Care Independent Study Course, Veterans Health Initiative: vaww.sites.lrn.va.gov/vhi (available through VA intranet only)
- National Center for PTSD website: www.ptsd.va.gov/professional/index.asp
- National Institute for Mental Health information on PTSD: www.nimh.nih.gov/health/topics/post-traumatic-stress-disorder-ptsd/index.shtml

# 4

# Depression

Service members and their families experience unique emotional challenges.

Deployment and redeployment, single parenting, and long absences of loved ones are a stressful part of military life. At times, these events can lead to sadness, feelings of hopelessness, and withdrawal from friends, families, and colleagues. Parenting can feel more a burden than a joy. We may feel irritable and even neglectful of our children's needs. When these feelings and behaviors appear, depression may be present. Seeking care for depression, for ourselves or loved ones, takes energy and courage.

## What Is It?

We all experience sadness or feel down from time to time. That's a normal part of being human. Depression, however, is different. It lasts longer and is more serious than normal sadness or grief. Common symptoms include:

Feeling down or sad more days than not
Losing interest in hobbies or activities that you used to find enjoyable or fun
Being excessively low in energy and/or overly tired
Feeling that things are never going to get better

Depression is one of the most common and treatable mental disorders. Delay in identifying depression often leads to needless suffering for the depressed individual and his or her family. Depression is not uncommon during or after the holiday season. Preparing for the holidays, the increased expectations of family and friends, the sadness of not having a loved one present, or having to say good-bye after a holiday reunion can contribute to depression.

## The Extent of the Problem

Depression is a common problem in which severe and long lasting feelings of sadness or other problems get in the way of a person's ability to function. In any given year, as many as 18.8 million American adults—9.5 percent of the adult population—experience some type of depression.

Unlike a blue mood that comes and goes, depression is a persistent problem that affects the way a person eats and sleeps, thinks about things, and feels about him- or herself.

## How Does It manifest Itself?

The symptoms of depression can vary quite a bit, but most people who experience depression feel down or sad more days than not, or find that things in their life no longer seem enjoyable or interesting.

*Symptoms of Adult Depression*

Persistent sad or empty mood
Loss of interest or pleasure in ordinary activities
Changes in appetite or sleep
Decreased energy or fatigue
Inability to concentrate, make decisions
Feelings of guilt, hopelessness or worthlessness
Thoughts of death or suicide

Additionally, people with depression may notice changes in their sleeping, eating, concentration, or feelings about themselves, and may find themselves feeling hopeless. These symptoms typically last for at least 2 weeks without letting up.

## Behavior and Depression

*Negative Action, Negative Mood*

People with the blues usually feel "down," tired, sad, and hopeless. The natural instinct when feeling down is to just go with the feelings. A person who is depressed might:

- Not do things that take energy or effort
- Decide that they will put things they don't want to do off until later when they feel better

- Keep to oneself and not spend time with family or friends
- Sleep a lot or spend a lot of time trying to sleep
- Misuse alcohol and other substances (such as, drugs, nicotine, or caffeine)
- Overeat, or not eat enough or nutritiously
- Avoid feelings or others by keeping busy with habit-forming activities such as watching television or video-gaming

Here's an interesting point about depression: when a person just goes with depressed feelings and stays away from activities, it is those very activities that are being avoided that may help a person to feel better. Not doing things only makes the depression worse because avoiding activities:

- Keeps a person from having fun and living a full life
- Puts off facing and solving problems
- Keeps a person from dealing with important feelings and issues (for example, grief when a loved one dies)
- Makes it harder to cope with painful feelings in the future
- Makes it more likely that the problems will get worse

## What Causes Depression?

Depression has many causes. Difficulty coping with painful experiences or losses contributes to depression. People returning from a war zone often experience painful memories, feelings of guilt, or regret about their war experiences, or have a tough time readjusting back to normal life.

Trouble coping with these feelings and experiences can lead to depression. Some types of depression run in families, and depression is often associated with chemical imbalances and other changes in the brain.

Depression is an illness that involves one's body, mood, and thoughts. It affects the way a person eats and sleeps, the way one feels about oneself, and the way one thinks about things. Depression is not a passing blue mood, nor is it a sign of personal weakness. Depression is a *medical* illness and a *treatable* illness just like diabetes or heart disease.

Individuals who are depressed often experience more difficulty in performing their job, caring for their children, and in their personal relationships.

A family history of depression and negative life experiences such as loss, trauma, serious illness, and stress can also contribute to the onset of depression. There are effective treatments today for depression including medications and therapy. Without treatment, symptoms can last for weeks, months, or years. Appropriate treatment, however, can help most people who suffer from depression.

## What Are the Treatment Options?

Depression is very treatable. Depression can be a part of chronic fatigue or unexplained aches and pains. The earlier depression is detected and treated, the less likely it is to develop into a more serious problem that can impact one's job, career, health, and relationships.

An evaluation should be done by a health care professional to help determine which type of treatment is best for an individual. Typically, milder forms of depression are treated by psychotherapy, and more severe depression is treated with medications or a combination of psychotherapy and medication. Your doctor can help you determine which treatment is best for you.

### *Psychotherapy*

There are a number of types of psychotherapy (or talk therapy) that are used to treat depression. These treatments may involve just a few sessions, or may last ten to twenty weeks or longer. Psychotherapy treatments tend to focus on helping patients learn about their problems and resolve them, through working with a therapist and learning new patterns of behavior to help decrease depression. Two of the main types of psychotherapy for depression are interpersonal therapy and cognitive-behavioral therapy. Interpersonal therapy focuses on the patient's relationships with other people, and how these relationships may cause and maintain depression.

Cognitive-behavioral treatments help patients change negative styles of thinking and acting that can lead to depression.

### *Medication*

In addition to psychotherapy, there are several types of antidepressant medications used to treat depression. These include selective serotonin reuptake inhibitors (SSRIs), tricyclics, and monoamine oxidase inhibitors (MAOIs). The newer medications for treating depression, such as the SSRIs, generally have fewer side effects than older types of medications. A health care provider may try more than one type of medication, or may increase the dosage, to find a treatment that works. Improvements in symptoms of depression typically occur after the medication is taken regularly for three to four weeks, although in some medications it may take as long as eight weeks for the full effect to occur.

Antidepressant medications are typically safe and effective. They help patients feel less depressed and generally do not make people feel "drugged" or different during their daily lives. The side effects of depression medications vary depending on the medication, and can include dry mouth, constipation, bladder problems, sexual problems, blurred vision, dizziness, drowsiness, headache, nausea, nervousness, or insomnia. Because of side effects or because they begin feeling better, patients are often tempted to stop taking their medication too soon. Some medications must be stopped slowly to give your body time to readjust to not having the medication. Never stop taking an antidepressant without consulting your doctor.

## How Can Family and Friends Assist in the Healing Process

*What Can I Do about Feelings of Depression?*

Depression can make a person feel exhausted, worthless, helpless, hopeless, and sad. These feelings can make you feel as though you are never going to feel better, or that you should just give up. It is important to realize that these negative thoughts and feelings are part of depression, and often fade as treatment begins working. In the meantime, here is a list of things to try to improve your mood:

- Talk with your doctor or health care provider.
- Talk with family and friends, and let them help you.
- Participate in activities that make you feel better, or that you used to enjoy before you began feeling depressed.
- Set realistic goals for yourself.
- Engage in mild exercise.
- Try to be with others and get support from them.
- Break up goals and tasks into smaller, more reachable ones.

## Resources Available

National Institute of Mental Health Depression Fact Sheet: www.nimh.nih.gov/publicat/depression.cfm
National Alliance for the Mentally Ill: www.nami.org
National Center for Posttraumatic Stress Disorder: www.ptsd.va.gov

# 5

# Anger

## What Is It?

Anger can sometimes turn into violence or physical abuse. It can also result in emotional and/or verbal abuse that can damage relationships. Abuse can take the form of threats, swearing, criticism, throwing things, conflict, pushing, grabbing, and hitting. If you were abused as a child, you are more at risk for abusing your partner or family members.

## The Extent of the Problem

Veterans of Operation Iraqi Freedom (OIF) who suffer from symptoms of posttraumatic stress disorder (PTSD) are likely to have difficulties with anger regulation given the centrality of anger in the human survival response.

Research among military veterans has consistently shown that those with PTSD are higher in anger, hostility, aggression, general violence, and relationship violence and abuse than those without the disorder (e.g., Jordan et al. 1992). "Irritability and outbursts of anger" represent one of the diagnostic criteria for PTSD (American Psychiatric Association 1994) and can have a debilitating impact across several domains. Anger dysregulation typically has a deleterious impact on the veteran's relationships with family members and other loved ones, and may significantly interfere with other social and occupational functioning. These interpersonal difficulties may have a profound negative effect on the veteran's social support network, which places him or her at risk for PTSD exacerbation, and possibly for cardiovascular disease and other health problems that have been associated with anger, hostility, and PTSD. Angry outbursts may also place the veteran at risk for legal problems and may lead to severe consequences for those who are exposed to these outbursts.

Although little theory or research explicates the role of PTSD with respect to anger, one important theory for anger problems among veterans with PTSD emphasizes the role of context-inappropriate activation of cognitive processes related to a "survival mode" of functioning (Chemtob et al. 1997).

This response includes heightened arousal, a hostile appraisal of events, loss of the ability to engage in self-monitoring or other inhibitory processes, and resulting behavior produced to respond to this perceived severe threat. These processes lead the veteran to see threats in the civilian environment that do not objectively pose any significant danger, and he or she may respond in an aggressive manner to such threats. This "survival mode," while adaptive in combat situations, typically becomes maladaptive when the individual interacts with his or her environment in civilian life. Therefore, in therapy with this population, an important treatment target often involves the detection of cognitive biases with respect to environmental threats and the detection of disconfirming evidence. This sense of heightened threat may be particularly acute among individuals who served in OIF because the enemy was not always clearly defined and military personnel were forced to be vigilant to attack at all times.

## How Does It Manifest Itself?

Here are a few warning signs that may lead to domestic violence:

Controlling behaviors or jealousy
Blaming others for problems or conflict
Radical mood changes
Verbal abuse such as humiliating, manipulating, confusing
Self-destructive or overly risky actions; heated arguments

### *Domestic Violence*

Domestic violence happens so much in the military that the Department of Defense (DoD) has made it an item of specific concern. First sergeants and military police hate domestic call-outs because the solutions are never clear cut. More often than not, the victims of domestic violence refuse to cooperate because they perceive a threat to their spouse's career. Understanding domestic violence, knowing the warning signs and what you can do, and how to get help are steps to help end this problem.

## UNDERSTANDING DOMESTIC VIOLENCE

Understanding domestic violence starts with understanding intimate partner violence (IPV). IPV happens when a current or former spouse or boyfriend / girlfriend stalks, harms, or threatens to harm their partner, physically, emotionally, or sexually. In addition, IPV is sometimes referred to as "domestic violence," a term that refers to any violence among family members. Individuals who have experienced IPV may have many health problems beyond any immediate physical injury, including:

- Depression
- Anxiety
- PTSD
- Suicide attempts
- Substance abuse
- Gastrointestinal disorders
- Sexually transmitted diseases
- Gynecological or pregnancy complications

Individuals who have experienced or are experiencing IPV may have a hard time keeping a job. They may also have trouble with their finances and the ability to support themselves or their children.

IPV is not gender specific. Both men and women can be victims of IPV. However, women, especially younger women, are most likely to be at risk. National surveys indicate that one in four women experience physical or sexual IPV in their lifetime. IPV can occur in both same-sex and opposite-sex relationships.

Research suggests IPV may happen more often among military service members and veterans than civilians. Stress and PTSD may increase the risk for IPV in some veteran relationships. One survey found that 24 percent of female Veterans Administration (VA) patients under age fifty experienced IPV in the past year.

The good news is that there are VA programs aimed at addressing the health effects of IPV and reducing IPV risk. For example, VA is researching and developing several IPV-intervention programs, including a couples-based therapy program. The VA is also researching and developing better ways to ask about IPV in primary care settings.

There are many types of talk therapies, which may help those who have experienced IPV deal with PTSD, depression, and anxiety. Some of these therapies, such as cognitive-processing therapy, are available to veterans through VA and at Vet Centers. They are there to help men and women with safety planning and locating services. Plus, every VA medical center has a Women Veterans Program Manager who can help.

KNOW THE WARNING SIGNS

- My partner has injured me badly enough that I needed medical attention.
- My partner follows me everywhere I go or needs to know what I am doing at all times.
- My partner has threatened to hurt my children or pets.
- My partner abuses alcohol or drugs.
- My partner has forced me to have sex.
- My partner has threatened to kill me.
- My partner has threatened to kill himself/herself.
- My partner has a gun or can get a gun easily.
- My partner is violent toward other people.
- My partner destroys my belongings.
- My partner controls my money.
- My partner tells me who I can spend time with.
- My partner calls me harsh names and makes me feel worthless.

**WHAT YOU CAN DO**

*Build Independence*

- Start saving money and store it in a safe place, such as a separate bank account.
- Talk to your VA health care provider about what is going on.
- Get help from a counselor, a health care provider, or legal services.
- Keep in touch with a trustworthy friend or family member.

*Be Prepared*

- Keep a little cash with you.
- Keep your cell phone charged and with you.
- Teach your children to go to a safe place (a friend's, neighbor's, or relative's home).
- Keep an emergency bag ready with
  - Medications/prescriptions
  - Phone card/change for pay phones
  - Extra keys
  - Bank card/credit cards
  - Custody order
  - Work permits
  - Photos of abuser
  - Address book
  - Your child's favorite toys
  - Money

- Cell phone and charger
- Photo ID / driver's license
- Restraining order
- Passports / immigration papers / green cards
- Electronic Benefit Transfer (EBT) card
- Clothes
- Toiletries and diapers

### HOW TO GET HELP

In addition to VA programs, there are community resources to help individuals who have experienced IPV. National and local hotlines can connect those who have experienced IPV with local shelters and programs where they can find safety and support.

- In an emergency you should call 911.
- National Domestic Violence Hotline 1-800-799-SAFE (7233)
- National Sexual Assault Hotline 1-800-656-HOPE (4673)
- National Suicide Hotline 1-800-SUICIDE (784-2433)

### LEARN MORE

- Understanding Intimate Partner Violence, US Centers for Disease Control and Prevention
- Preventing Intimate Partner and Sexual Violence: Program Activities Guide, US Centers for Disease Control and Prevention

### COURSES OF ACTION

In most cases, husbands abuse wives, but that's not always true. If the abuser is a civilian, the military has no control over the matter. In most cases, all the military can do is turn the information over to civilian authorities. Installation commanders do have the power to bar civilians from military installations, and will exercise that power to protect military members from abusive civilian spouses, if necessary.

If the abuser is a military member, domestic violence situations are handled on two separate tracks: the military justice system, and the Family Advocacy system. It's important to realize that these are two separate systems, not connected. Family advocacy is an identification, intervention, and treatment program—not a punishment system. It's entirely possible that the Family Advocacy Committee will return a finding of "substantiated abuse," but there will be insufficient legally admissible evidence to allow punishment under the provisions of military justice.

On the other hand, one should realize that the Family Advocacy system does not enjoy the right of "confidentiality" under military law (such as chaplains and attorneys), and evidence gathered and statements made during Family Advocacy investigations may be used in military justice proceedings.

If the incident(s) happen off base, civilian agencies may be given jurisdiction on the legal side, but Family Advocacy should still be notified. Off base, local police may or may not report the incident to base officials. DoD officials are currently working to develop memoranda of understanding with civilian law-enforcement authorities to establish such reporting procedures.

Regulations require military and DoD officials to report any suspicion of family violence to Family Advocacy, no matter how small. This includes commanders, first sergeants, supervisors, medical personnel, teachers, and military police.

In many cases, when responding to a domestic situation, the commander or first sergeant will order the military individual to reside in the dormitory/barracks until the Family Advocacy investigation is completed. This may be accompanied by a "military protective order," which is a written order prohibiting the military member from having any contact with the alleged victim. Many bases have an "abused dependent safeguard" system, where the first sergeant or commander can place the family members in billeting under an assumed name.

When domestic violence is reported to Family Advocacy, the agency will assign a caseworker to assess the victim's safety, develop a safety plan, and investigate the incident. Throughout the process, victims' advocates ensure that the victim's medical, mental health, and protection needs are being met. Family Advocacy officials will also interview the alleged abuser. The alleged abuser is informed of his or her rights under the provisions of Article 31 of the Uniform Code of Military Justice (UCMJ), and does not have to speak to the investigation officials, if he or she chooses not to.

If child abuse is involved, regulations require that local child-protection agencies be notified, and participate in the process.

After the investigation, the case is then presented to a multidisciplinary case-review committee with representatives from the Family Advocacy Program, law enforcement, staff judge advocate, medical staff, and chaplain. The committee decides whether the evidence indicates abuse occurred, and arrives at one of the following findings:

*Substantiated.* A case that has been investigated and the preponderance of available information indicates that abuse has occurred. This means that the information that supports the occurrence of abuse is of greater weight or more convincing than the information that indicates that abuse did not occur.

*Suspected.* A case determination is pending further investigation. Duration for a case to be "suspected" and under investigation should not exceed twelve weeks.

*Unsubstantiated.* An alleged case that has been investigated and the available information is insufficient to support the claim that child abuse and/or neglect or spouse abuse did occur. The family needs no family advocacy services.

In making these determinations, the committee uses the following definitions for abuse:

*Child Abuse and/or Neglect.* Includes physical injury, sexual maltreatment, emotional maltreatment, deprivation of necessities, or combinations for a child by an individual responsible for the child's welfare under circumstances indicating that the child's welfare is harmed or threatened. The term encompasses both acts and omissions on the part of a responsible person. A "child" is a person under eighteen years of age for whom a parent, guardian, foster parent, caretaker, employee of a residential facility, or any staff person providing out-of-home care is legally responsible. The term "child" means a natural child, adopted child, stepchild, foster child, or ward. The term also includes an individual of any age who is incapable for self-support because of a mental or physical incapacity and for whom treatment in a Military Treatment Facility (MTF) is authorized.

*Spouse Abuse.* Includes assault, battery, threat to injure or kill, other act of force or violence, or emotional maltreatment inflicted on a partner in a lawful marriage when one of the partners is a military member or is employed by the DoD and is eligible for treatment in an MTF. A spouse under eighteen years of age shall be treated in this category.

Based on the committee's recommendations, the commander decides what action to take regarding the abuser. The commander determines whether to order the individual into treatment, and/or to seek to impose disciplinary procedures under the Uniform Code of Military Justice. The commander may also seek to obtain the discharge of the service member from the military.

Victims often hesitate to report abuse because they fear the impact it will have on their spouse's career. A recent DoD study found that service members reported for abuse are 23 percent more likely to be separated from the service than nonabusers and somewhat more likely to have other than honorable discharges. The majority who remain in the military are more likely to be promoted more slowly than nonabusers.

Many military spouses don't know that federal law gives financial protection to the spouse if the member is discharged for an offense which "*involves abuse of the then-current spouse or a dependent child.*" It doesn't matter if the discharge is a punitive discharge imposed by a court-martial, or an administrative discharge initiated by the commander. The key is that the reason for the discharge must be for a "dependent abuse" offense.

The term "involves abuse of the then-current spouse or a dependent child" means that the criminal offense is against the person of that spouse or a dependent child. Crimes that may qualify as "dependent-abuse offenses" are ones such as sexual assault, rape, sodomy, assault, battery, murder, and manslaughter.

You can check to see what the current authorized payment is. If the spouse has custody of a dependent child or children of the member, the amount of monthly compensation is increased for each child. If there is no eligible spouse, compensation paid to a dependent child or children is paid in equal shares to each child.

The duration of the payments cannot exceed thirty-six months. If the military member had less than thirty-six months of obligated military service at the time of the discharge or imposition of the court-martial sentence, then the duration of the payments is the length of the member's obligated service, or twelve months, whichever is greater.

If a spouse receiving payments remarries, payments terminate as of the date of the remarriage. Payment is not to be renewed if such remarriage is terminated. If the payments to the spouse terminate due to remarriage and there is a dependent child not living in the same household as the spouse or member, payments are be made to the dependent child.

If the military member who committed the abuse resides in the same household as the spouse or dependent child to whom compensation is otherwise payable, payment terminates as of the date the member begins residing in such household.

If the victim was a dependent child, and the spouse has been found by competent authority designated by the Secretary concerned to have been an active participant in the conduct constituting the criminal offense or to have actively aided or abetted the member in such conduct against that dependent child, the spouse, a dependent child living with the spouse is not to be paid transitional compensation.

In addition to the transitional benefits, if the military member was eligible for retirement, and was denied retirement because of the criminal offense, the spouse can still apply to a divorce court for a division of retired pay under the provisions of the Uniformed Services Former Spouse Protection Act, and the military will honor the payments. (Note: Under this provision, such payments terminate upon remarriage.)

Even if a domestic violence case is handled off base via the civilian criminal court system, criminal conviction of even a misdemeanor involving domestic violence can end a service member's military career. The 1996 Lautenberg Amendment to the Gun Control Act of 1968 makes it unlawful for anyone who has been convicted of a misdemeanor of domestic violence to possess firearms. The law applies to law enforcement officers and military personnel.

## HOW CAN FAMILY AND FRIENDS ASSIST?

An excellent way for families to communicate is through regular family meetings (Fetsch and Jacobson 2007). This can enhance moral reasoning and manage anger long before it turns into violence. Regular family meetings can promote family harmony by providing a safe time and place for making decisions, recognizing good things happening in the family, setting up rules, distributing chores fairly, settling conflicts, and pointing out individual strengths.

Some families are ready for self-directed enrichment and problem solving like that recommended here. Other families first need family or marriage therapy because their situations are too troubled to be worked out without professional assistance. To help assess whether your family is ready to try family meetings, answer the following questions:

- Are we as parents committed to using words and communication to solve problems as a family?
- Can we as a family discuss issues and differences without screaming, yelling, and fighting?
- Do we at least sometimes listen to and hear one another's viewpoints?

If you answered yes to most of these questions, then read on and try the steps below. Otherwise, ask your friends for the names of therapists who are effective at assisting families who have situations similar to yours. Look in the yellow pages of your telephone book under counselors and make an appointment to seek the professional assistance your family needs.

If a formal family meeting does not seem workable in your family at the present time, work toward this end by planning to eat meals together. Use this time to share the day's happenings and celebrate successes of family members. Involve the whole family in planning, rather than having just parents plan for holidays, vacations, and weekend outings. When a controversy develops with another family member, have a discussion.

Use good problem-solving skills. Identify the specific problem you want to solve and talk about the possible ways to solve it. Talk about the pros and cons of each solution and come to an agreement about the best one. When this way of problem solving feels comfortable, gradually involve other family members. Compliment children when you hear them solving their problems using the skills you have taught them.

When your family is ready, begin planning formal meetings. Set aside time to be together and to look at your lives and what works and what does not.

Begin with an attitude of openness and acceptance rather than one of dominance or control. Be flexible. The meeting place and length can vary. At first, plan fun activities that involve everybody: "Let's have a family meeting soon to talk about your birthday. Is Sunday after supper a good time for you?"

Set a date and time when all family members can be there. An elderly family member living in the home may also be invited. Invite everybody but don't require them to be present. The consequence of not being present is that their views will be missing as the family makes decisions that may affect them.

As soon as children can use words, they can participate. Especially with young children (ages two to six), keep the family meeting as short as ten to twenty minutes, gradually increasing the time. With older children, decide ahead how much time to allow.

Many families find it valuable to schedule meetings for the same time and place every week or every other week. Design the meetings to fit the family. Intergenerational families sometimes find monthly meetings better.

The length is determined by the topics to be discussed. By holding family meetings regularly, it is easier to keep them balanced to both celebrate happy times and solve family problems. Discussing one or two problems per meeting usually is a good limit.

*Tips for Successful Family Meetings* The purpose of a family meeting is to foster open communication among family members. It is a safe place where everyone is free to say what they think and feel as they cooperate to make decisions and solve problems. A structured meeting helps this to happen when a family is ready for it.

1. Meet at a regularly scheduled time.

   Begin and end on time. Guard meeting times and encourage high commitment by keeping them a high priority.

2. Rotate meeting responsibilities, e.g., leader, secretary, and timekeeper.

   Treating everybody as equals provides all family members with practice at problem solving. Encourage all to be good listeners. The original leader should be an adult family member who believes in equal rights and democratic relationships. The leader starts and ends the meeting on time and helps the family develop the rules to follow. One example of a rule is: only one person speaks at a time; the rest listen well enough so they can repeat back to the speaker's satisfaction what he or she said and feels. The leader makes sure all points of view are heard.

   The leader also keeps the communication focused on one topic at a time and ends the meeting on time. At the end of the meeting, the family decides who will be the leader, secretary, and timekeeper next time. Some families choose to have a secretary who keeps minutes of decisions and agreements. The secretary also can record activities and deadlines on a calendar for all to see. The next meeting can begin with a recap by the secretary. The minutes can be a family journal that is kept to look back on in later years. The roles of leader and secretary can be rotated among the adults until everyone feels at ease with how to conduct an effective family meeting. Then these roles can be rotated among younger children as well.

3. Encourage all family members to participate.

   In a safe environment, family members can express their opinions without punishment or retaliation. Show lots of love. Some parents are just beginning to experiment with shifting from an authoritarian to an authoritative parenting style. At first, they sometimes feel more comfortable limiting open discussion to smaller issues with less serious consequences. These parents are encouraged not to worry too much and let logical consequences of less serious actions speak for themselves.

4. Discuss one topic and solve one problem at a time.

   "The problem we want to solve today is . . . I suggest we devote . . . minutes to this issue. Is this agreeable?" Later the family can renegotiate more time if necessary. As the leader notices the discussion moving off track, he or she might say: "That sounds like an issue we may want to discuss at another time. But for now the issue we're here to discuss is. . . ." As the leader notices someone interrupting the speaker, he or she might say: "Excuse me, _____. We want to hear your opinion—it is important to us. Could you hold it until _____ is finished talking?"

5. Use I-messages and problem-solving steps. For information about how to create I-messages, see fact sheet 10.236, *Dealing with Our Anger* at www.ext.colostate.edu/pubs/consumer/10236.html. For problem-solving steps, see fact sheet 10.238, *Dealing with Couples' Anger* at www.ext.colostate.edu/pubs/consumer/10238.html.

6. Summarize the discussion to keep the family on track and to focus the discussion on one issue at a time.

   Summarize the current agreement as necessary. Look for nonverbal and verbal signs that a family member is uncomfortable with something.

7. Make decisions by consensus.

   Consensus is defined as communicating, problem-solving, and negotiating on major issues until no family member has any major objections to the decision—all can live with it. Autocratic decision making allows one person to decide. Democratic decision making allows the majority to decide. Neither works well in families where people live, work, and play side by side. Those family members who do not feel heard may sabotage decisions made this way. Decision making by consensus incorporates the major needs and wants of all. It allows effective communication, problem solving, anger, and conflict management.

8. Once it appears that you have an agreement, make sure you have reached consensus.

   "What I'm hearing us say we can all agree to do is. . . . Does anyone have any major objections?" If someone does, talk and negotiate some more.

9. If things get "too hot to handle," anyone can call for a break.

   Take a break for perhaps fifteen minutes, or whatever time is needed, before meeting again.

10. End with something that is fun and that affirms family members.

    Enjoy a family tradition, a bowl of popcorn, and a good television program, or a game that everybody enjoys.

*Evaluate and Adjust* Remember, just as family members grow and change over time, so, too, do rules for family meetings.

If children want to do something that seems like a mistake, discuss it rather than lay down the law or forbid it. Raise some of the issues or consequences they may have overlooked. If the matter is not too serious, it might be a good learning experience for them to deal with these consequences, especially if parents can teach in a coaching rather than a blaming manner. Children are more apt to learn to make good decisions if they have full knowledge ahead of time and then assume responsibility for decisions, both good and bad.

To evaluate your family's progress, assess how well the children take responsibility for problem solving. Do any family members feel closer to each other? Is the trust level increasing? Noticing small positive changes is a good way to encourage continued progress. Slagle (1985) offers additional practical ideas for conducting effective family meetings.

If your family just cannot seem to find a time when everybody can get together and talk, adapt the steps in this fact sheet. Consider alternatives. Perhaps you can touch base with your spouse and children individually on how they are doing, which decisions need to be made alone, and which need to be made together. Stopping periodically to discuss decisions that relate to all family members, scribbling dates on the calendar, and talking on the run may be the best you can do under the circumstances.

The key to successful family meetings is to be flexible. Use what works to help your family ride the ups and downs of family living and to bounce back after a stressful event. Families that know how to adapt well to inevitable changes tend to have higher marital and family satisfaction levels.

# 6

# ANXIETY

## What Is It?

Anxiety is a generalized mood condition that can occur without an identifiable triggering stimulus. As such, it is distinguished from fear, which is an appropriate cognitive and emotional response to a perceived threat. Additionally, fear is related to the specific behaviors of escape and avoidance, whereas anxiety is related to situations perceived as uncontrollable or unavoidable.

Another view defines anxiety as "a future-oriented mood state in which one is ready or prepared to attempt to cope with upcoming negative events," suggesting that it is a distinction between future and present dangers that divides anxiety and fear. In a 2011 review of the literature by Sylvers, Lilienfeld, and Laprarie in the *Clinical Psychology Review*, fear and anxiety were said to be differentiated in four domains: (1) duration of emotional experience, (2) temporal focus, (3) specificity of the threat, and (4) motivated direction. Fear was defined as short lived, present focused, geared toward a specific threat, and facilitating escape from threat; while anxiety was defined as long acting, future focused, broadly focused toward a diffuse threat, and promoting caution while approaching a potential threat.

The psychologist David H. Barlow of Boston University conducted a study (2002) that showed three common characteristics of people suffering from chronic anxiety, which he characterized as "a generalized biological vulnerability," "a generalized psychological vulnerability," and "a specific psychological vulnerability." While chemical issues in the brain that result in anxiety (especially resulting from genetics) are well documented, this study highlights an additional environmental factor that may result from being raised by parents suffering from chronic anxiety themselves.

People who experience anxiety disorders have excessive worry, tension, fearfulness, or uncertainty. The anxiety causes significant distress or impairment in their ability to function in some area of their lives. Anxiety disorders often occur with other physical or mental disorders. Some people with anxiety experience panic attacks. A panic attack is a period of intense fear or discomfort without real danger. There are many other symptoms that can occur when someone experiences a panic attack.

## The Extent of the Problem

Anxiety disorders affect about forty million American adults age eighteen years and older (about 18 percent) in a given year, causing them to be filled with fearfulness and uncertainty. Unlike the relatively mild, brief anxiety caused by a stressful event (such as speaking in public or a first date), anxiety disorders last at least six months and can get worse if they are not treated. Anxiety disorders commonly occur along with other mental or physical illnesses, including alcohol or substance abuse, which may mask anxiety symptoms or make them worse. In some cases, these other illnesses need to be treated before a person will respond to treatment for the anxiety disorder.

## How Does It Manifest Itself?

Anxiety can be a symptom of an underlying health issue such as chronic obstructive pulmonary disease (COPD), heart failure, or heart arrythmia.

Abnormal and pathological anxiety or fear may itself be a medical condition falling under the blanket term "anxiety disorder." Such conditions came under the aegis of psychiatry at the end of the nineteenth century and current psychiatric diagnostic criteria recognize several specific forms of the disorder. Recent surveys have found that as many as 18 percent of Americans may be affected by one or more of them.

Standardized screening tools such as Zung Self-Rating Anxiety Scale, Beck Anxiety Inventory, and Hamilton Anxiety Scale (HAM-A) can be used to detect anxiety symptoms and suggest the need for a formal diagnostic assessment of anxiety disorder. The HAM-A measures the severity of a patient's anxiety, based on fourteen parameters, including anxious mood, tension, fears, insomnia, somatic complaints, and behavior at the interview.

Overwhelming anxiety, if not treated early, can consequently become a generalized anxiety disorder (GAD), which can be identified by symptoms of exaggerated and excessive worry, chronic anxiety, and constant, irrational thoughts. The anxious thoughts and feelings felt while suffering from GAD are difficult to control and can cause serious mental anguish that interferes with normal, daily functioning.

The Diagnostic and Statistical Manual of Mental Disorders (DSM-IV) includes specific criteria for diagnosing generalized anxiety disorder. The DSM-IV states that a patient must experience chronic anxiety and excessive worry, almost daily, for at least six months due to a number of stressors (such as work or school) and experience three or more defined symptoms, including, "restlessness or feeling keyed up or on edge, being easily fatigued, difficulty concentrating or mind going blank, irritability, muscle tension, sleep disturbance (difficulty falling or staying asleep, or restless unsatisfying sleep)."

If symptoms of chronic anxiety are not addressed and treated in adolescence then the risk of developing an anxiety disorder in adulthood increases significantly. "Clinical worry is also associated with risk of comorbidity with other anxiety disorders and depression" which is why immediate treatment is so important.

GAD can be treated through specialized therapies aimed at changing thinking patterns and in turn reducing anxiety-producing behaviors. Cognitive behavioral therapy (CBT) and short-term psychodynamic psychotherapy (STPP) can be used to successfully treat GAD with positive effects lasting twelve months after treatment. There are also other treatment plans that should be discussed with a knowledgeable health care practitioner, which can be used in conjunction with behavioral therapy to greatly reduce the disabling symptoms of GAD.

Anxiety can be either a short-term "state" or a long-term "trait." Trait anxiety reflects a stable tendency to respond with state anxiety in the anticipation of threatening situations. It is closely related to the personality trait of neuroticism. Such anxiety may be conscious or unconscious.

The physical effects of anxiety may include heart palpitations, tachycardia, muscle weakness and tension, fatigue, nausea, chest pain, shortness of breath, stomach aches, or headaches. As the body prepares to deal with a threat, blood pressure, heart rate, perspiration, and blood flow to the major muscle groups are increased, while immune and digestive functions are inhibited (the *fight-or-flight* response). External signs of anxiety may include pallor, sweating, trembling, and pupillary dilation. Someone who has anxiety might also experience it subjectively as a sense of dread or panic.

Although panic attacks are not experienced by every person who has anxiety, they are a common symptom. Panic attacks usually come without warning and although the fear is generally irrational, the subjective perception of danger is very real. A person experiencing a panic attack will often feel as if he or she is about to die or lose consciousness.

The **emotional effects** of anxiety may include "feelings of apprehension or dread, trouble concentrating, feeling tense or jumpy, anticipating the worst, irritability, restlessness, watching (and waiting) for signs (and occurrences) of danger, and, feeling like your mind's gone blank" as well as "nightmares/bad dreams, obsessions about sensations, deja vu, a trapped in your mind feeling, and feeling like everything is scary."

The cognitive effects of anxiety may include thoughts about suspected dangers, such as fear of dying. "You may . . . fear that the chest pains are a deadly heart attack or that the shooting pains in your head are the result of a tumor or aneurysm. You feel an intense fear when you think of dying, or you may think of it more often than normal, or can't get it out of your mind."

The behavioral effects of anxiety may include withdrawal from situations that have provoked anxiety in the past. Anxiety can also be experienced in ways that include changes in sleeping patterns, nervous habits, and increased motor tension like foot tapping.

The following are anxiety disorders:

- Generalized anxiety disorder (GAD)
- Social phobia
- Obsessive-compulsive disorder (OCD)
- Posttraumatic stress disorder (PTSD)
- Panic disorder
- Specific phobias
- Agoraphobia

Panic disorder is a real illness that can be successfully treated. It is characterized by sudden attacks of terror, usually accompanied by a pounding heart, sweatiness, weakness, faintness, or dizziness. During these attacks, people with panic disorder may flush or feel chilled; their hands may tingle or feel numb; and they may experience nausea, chest pain, or smothering sensations. Panic attacks usually produce a sense of unreality, a fear of impending doom, or a fear of losing control.

A fear of one's own unexplained physical symptoms is also a symptom of panic disorder. People having panic attacks sometimes believe they are having heart attacks, losing their minds, or on the verge of death. They can't predict when or where an attack will occur, and between episodes many worry intensely and dread the next attack.

Panic attacks can occur at any time, even during sleep. An attack usually peaks within ten minutes, but some symptoms may last much longer.

Panic disorder affects about six million American adults and is twice as common in women as men. Panic attacks often begin in late adolescence or early adulthood, but not everyone who experiences panic attacks will develop panic disorder. Many people have just one attack and never have another. The tendency to develop panic attacks appears to be inherited.

People who have full-blown, repeated panic attacks can become very disabled by their condition and should seek treatment before they start to avoid places or situations where panic attacks have occurred. For example, if a panic attack happened in an elevator, someone with panic disorder may develop a fear of elevators that could affect the choice of a job or an apartment, and restrict where that person can seek medical attention or enjoy entertainment.

Some people's lives become so restricted that they avoid normal activities, such as grocery shopping or driving. About one-third become housebound or are able to confront a feared situation only when accompanied by a spouse or other trusted person. When the condition progresses this far, it is called agoraphobia, or fear of open spaces.

Early treatment can often prevent agoraphobia, but people with panic disorder may sometimes go from doctor to doctor for years and visit the emergency room repeatedly before someone correctly diagnoses their condition. This is unfortunate, because panic disorder is one of the most treatable of all the anxiety disorders, responding in most cases to certain kinds of medication or certain kinds of cognitive psychotherapy, which help change thinking patterns that lead to fear and anxiety.

People with obsessive compulsive disorder (OCD) have persistent, upsetting thoughts (obsessions) and use rituals (compulsions) to control the anxiety these thoughts produce. Most of the time, the rituals end up controlling them.

For example, if people are obsessed with germs or dirt, they may develop a compulsion to wash their hands over and over again. If they develop an obsession with intruders, they may lock and relock their doors many times before going to bed. Being afraid of social embarrassment may prompt people with OCD to comb their hair compulsively in front of a mirror—sometimes they get "caught" in the mirror and can't move away from it. Performing such rituals is not pleasurable. At best, it produces temporary relief from the anxiety created by obsessive thoughts.

Other common rituals are a need to repeatedly check things, touch things (especially in a particular sequence), or count things. Some common obsessions include having frequent thoughts of violence and harming loved ones, persistently thinking about performing sexual acts the person dislikes, or having thoughts that are prohibited by religious beliefs. People with OCD may also be preoccupied with order and symmetry, have difficulty throwing things out (so they accumulate), or hoard unneeded items.

Healthy people also have rituals, such as checking to see if the stove is off several times before leaving the house. The difference is that people with OCD perform their rituals even though doing so interferes with daily life and they find the repetition distressing. Although most adults with

OCD recognize that what they are doing is senseless, some adults and most children may not realize that their behavior is out of the ordinary.

OCD affects about 2.2 million American adults, and the problem can be accompanied by eating disorders, other anxiety disorders, or depression. It strikes men and women in roughly equal numbers and usually appears in childhood, adolescence, or early adulthood. One-third of adults with OCD develop symptoms as children, and research indicates that OCD might run in families.

The course of the disease is quite varied. Symptoms may come and go, ease over time, or get worse. If OCD becomes severe, it can keep a person from working or carrying out normal responsibilities at home. People with OCD may try to help themselves by avoiding situations that trigger their obsessions, or they may use alcohol or drugs to calm themselves.

OCD usually responds well to treatment with certain medications and/or exposure-based psychotherapy, in which people face situations that cause fear or anxiety and become less sensitive (desensitized) to them. National Institutes of Mental Health (NIMH) is supporting research into new treatment approaches for people whose OCD does not respond well to the usual therapies. These approaches include combination and augmentation (add-on) treatments, as well as modern techniques such as deep brain stimulation.

Social phobia, also called social anxiety disorder, is diagnosed when people become overwhelmingly anxious and excessively self-conscious in everyday social situations. People with social phobia have an intense, persistent, and chronic fear of being watched and judged by others and of doing things that will embarrass them. They can worry for days or weeks before a dreaded situation. This fear may become so severe that it interferes with work, school, and other ordinary activities, and can make it hard to make and keep friends.

While many people with social phobia realize that their fears about being with people are excessive or unreasonable, they are unable to overcome them. Even if they manage to confront their fears and be around others, they are usually very anxious beforehand, are intensely uncomfortable throughout the encounter, and worry about how they were judged for hours afterward.

Social phobia can be limited to one situation (such as talking to people, eating or drinking, or writing on a blackboard in front of others) or may be so broad (such as in generalized social phobia) that the person experiences anxiety around almost anyone other than the family.

Physical symptoms that often accompany social phobia include blushing, profuse sweating, trembling, nausea, and difficulty talking. When these symptoms occur, people with social phobia feel as though all eyes are focused on them.

Social phobia affects about fifteen million American adults. Women and men are equally likely to develop the disorder, which usually begins in childhood or early adolescence. There is some evidence that genetic factors are involved. Social phobia is often accompanied by other anxiety disorders or depression, and substance abuse may develop if people try to self-medicate their anxiety.

Social phobia can be successfully treated with certain kinds of psychotherapy or medications.

A specific phobia is an intense, irrational fear of something that actually poses little or no threat. Some of the more common specific phobias are heights, escalators, tunnels, highway driving, closed-in places, water, flying, dogs, spiders, and injuries involving blood. People with specific phobias may be able to ski the world's tallest mountains with ease but be unable to go above the fifth floor of an office building. While adults with phobias realize that these fears are irrational, they often find that facing, or even thinking about facing, the feared object or situation brings on a panic attack or severe anxiety.

Specific phobias affect around 19.2 million American adults and are twice as common in women as men. They usually appear in childhood or adolescence and tend to persist into adulthood. The causes of specific phobias are not well understood, but there is some evidence that the tendency to develop them may run in families.

If the feared situation or feared object is easy to avoid, people with specific phobias may not seek help; but if avoidance interferes with their careers or their personal lives, it can become disabling and treatment is usually pursued.

Specific phobias respond very well to carefully targeted psychotherapy.

People with GAD go through the day filled with exaggerated worry and tension, even though there is little or nothing to provoke it. They anticipate disaster and are overly concerned about health issues, money, family problems, or difficulties at work. Sometimes just the thought of getting through the day produces anxiety.

GAD is diagnosed when a person worries excessively about a variety of everyday problems for at least six months. People with GAD can't seem to get rid of their concerns, even though they usually realize that their anxiety is more intense than the situation warrants. They can't relax, startle easily, and have difficulty concentrating. Often they have trouble falling asleep or staying asleep. Physical symptoms that often accompany the anxiety include fatigue, headaches, muscle tension, muscle aches, difficulty swallowing, trembling, twitching, irritability, sweating, nausea, lightheadedness, having to go to the bathroom frequently, feeling out of breath, and hot flashes.

When their anxiety level is mild, people with GAD can function socially and hold down a job. Although they don't avoid certain situations as a result of their disorder, people with GAD can have difficulty carrying out the simplest daily activities if their anxiety is severe.

GAD affects about 6.8 million American adults, including twice as many women as men. The disorder develops gradually and can begin at any point in the life cycle, although the years of highest risk are between childhood and middle age. There is evidence that genes play a modest role in the disorder.

Other anxiety disorders, depression, or substance abuse often accompany GAD, which rarely occurs alone. GAD is commonly treated with medication or CBT, but co-occurring conditions must also be treated using the appropriate therapies.

## What Are the Treatment Options?

Treatments for anxiety disorders may include medication or therapy; both types have been found effective. A combination of medication and therapy may also be effective. The decision about treatment is based on your needs and preferences. Discuss your options with a professional who is familiar with your diagnosis and overall health. There is growing scientific evidence about complementary and alternative treatment, which is an approach to health care that exists outside conventional medicine practiced in the United States.

Consult a doctor or therapist to get a proper diagnosis and to learn about treatment options, length of treatment, side effects, time commitment, and other health issues to help you decide on the best treatment approach for you.

In general, anxiety disorders are treated with medication, specific types of psychotherapy, or both. Treatment choices depend on the problem and the person's preference. Before treatment begins, a doctor must conduct a careful diagnostic evaluation to determine whether a person's symptoms are caused by an anxiety disorder or a physical problem. If an anxiety disorder is diagnosed, the type of disorder or the combination of disorders that are present must be identified, as well as any coexisting conditions, such as depression or substance abuse. Sometimes alcoholism, depression, or other coexisting conditions have such a strong effect on the individual that treating the anxiety disorder must wait until the coexisting conditions are brought under control.

People with anxiety disorders who have already received treatment should tell their current doctor about that treatment in detail. If they received medication, they should tell their doctor what medication was used, what the dosage was at the beginning of treatment, whether the dosage was increased or decreased while they were under treatment, what side effects occurred, and whether the treatment helped them become less anxious. If they received psychotherapy, they should describe the type of therapy, how often they attended sessions, and whether the therapy was useful.

Often people believe that they have "failed" at treatment or that the treatment didn't work for them when, in fact, it was not given for an adequate length of time or was administered incorrectly. Sometimes people must try several different treatments or combinations of treatment before they find the one that works for them.

### *Medication*

Medication will not cure anxiety disorders, but it can keep them under control while the person receives psychotherapy. Medication must be prescribed by physicians, usually psychiatrists, who can either offer psychotherapy themselves or work as a team with psychologists, social workers, or counselors who provide psychotherapy. The principal medications used for anxiety disorders are antidepressants, antianxiety drugs, and beta-blockers to control some of the physical symptoms. With proper treatment, many people with anxiety disorders can lead normal, fulfilling lives.

#### ANTIDEPRESSANTS

Antidepressants were developed to treat depression but are also effective for anxiety disorders. Although these medications begin to alter brain chemistry after the very first dose, their full effect requires a series of changes to occur; it is usually about four to six weeks before symptoms start to fade. It is important to continue taking these medications long enough to let them work.

#### SEROTONIN REUPTAKE INHIBITORS (SSRIS)

Some of the newest antidepressants are called selective serotonin reuptake inhibitors, or SSRIs. SSRIs alter the levels of the neurotransmitter serotonin in the brain, which, like other neurotransmitters, helps brain cells communicate with one another.

Fluoxetine (Prozac®), sertraline (Zoloft®), escitalopram (Lexapro®), paroxetine (Paxil®), and citalopram (Celexa®) are some of the SSRIs commonly prescribed for panic disorder, OCD, PTSD, and social phobia. SSRIs are also used to treat panic disorder when it occurs in combination with OCD, social phobia, or depression. Venlafaxine (Effexor®), a drug closely related to the SSRIs, is used to treat GAD. These medications are started at low doses and gradually increased until they have a beneficial effect.

SSRIs have fewer side effects than older antidepressants, but they sometimes produce slight nausea or jitters when people first start to take them. These symptoms fade with time. Some people also experience sexual dysfunction with SSRIs, which may be helped by adjusting the dosage or switching to another SSRI.

### TRICYCLICS

Tricyclics are older than SSRIs and work as well as SSRIs for anxiety disorders other than OCD. They are also started at low doses that are gradually increased. They sometimes cause dizziness, drowsiness, dry mouth, and weight gain, which can usually be corrected by changing the dosage or switching to another tricyclic medication.

Tricyclics include imipramine (Tofranil®), which is prescribed for panic disorder and GAD, and clomipramine (Anafranil®), which is the only tricyclic antidepressant useful for treating OCD.

### MONOAMINE OXIDASE INHIBITORS (MAOIS)

Monoamine oxidase inhibitors (MAOIs) are the oldest class of antidepressant medications. The MAOIs most commonly prescribed for anxiety disorders are phenelzine (Nardil®), followed by tranylcypromine (Parnate®), and isocarboxazid (Marplan®), which are useful in treating panic disorder and social phobia. People who take MAOIs cannot eat a variety of foods and beverages (including cheese and red wine) that contain tyramine or take certain medications, including some types of birth control pills, pain relievers (such as Advil®, Motrin®, or Tylenol®), cold and allergy medications, and herbal supplements; these substances can interact with MAOIs to cause dangerous increases in blood pressure. The development of a new MAOI skin patch may help lessen these risks. MAOIs can also react with SSRIs to produce a serious condition called "serotonin syndrome," which can cause confusion, hallucinations, increased sweating, muscle stiffness, seizures, changes in blood pressure or heart rhythm, and other potentially life-threatening conditions.

### ANTIANXIETY DRUGS

High-potency benzodiazepines combat anxiety and have few side effects other than drowsiness. Because people can get used to them and may need higher and higher doses to get the same effect, benzodiazepines are generally prescribed for short periods of time, especially for people who have abused drugs or alcohol and who become dependent on medication easily. One exception to this rule is people with panic disorder, who can take benzodiazepines for up to a year without harm.

Clonazepam (Klonopin®) is used for social phobia and GAD, lorazepam (Ativan®) is helpful for panic disorder, and alprazolam (Xanax®) is useful for both panic disorder and GAD.

Some people experience withdrawal symptoms if they stop taking benzodiazepines abruptly instead of tapering off, and anxiety can return once the medication is stopped. These potential problems have led some physicians to shy away from using these drugs or to use them in inadequate doses.

Buspirone (Buspar®), an azapirone, is a newer antianxiety medication used to treat GAD. Possible side effects include dizziness, headaches, and nausea. Unlike benzodiazepines, buspirone must be taken consistently for at least two weeks to achieve an antianxiety effect.

#### BETA-BLOCKERS

Beta-blockers, such as propranolol (Inderal®), which is used to treat heart conditions, can prevent the physical symptoms that accompany certain anxiety disorders, particularly social phobia. When a feared situation can be predicted (such as giving a speech), a doctor may prescribe a beta-blocker to keep physical symptoms of anxiety under control.

### *Psychotherapy*

Psychotherapy involves talking with a trained mental health professional, such as a psychiatrist, psychologist, social worker, or counselor, to discover what caused an anxiety disorder and how to deal with its symptoms.

#### COGNITIVE BEHAVIORAL THERAPY (CBT)

CBT is very useful in treating anxiety disorders. The cognitive part helps people change the thinking patterns that support their fears, and the behavioral part helps people change the way they react to anxiety-provoking situations.

For example, CBT can help people with panic disorder learn that their panic attacks are not really heart attacks and help people with social phobia learn how to overcome the belief that others are always watching and judging them. When people are ready to confront their fears, they are shown how to use exposure techniques to desensitize themselves to situations that trigger their anxieties.

People with OCD who fear dirt and germs are encouraged to get their hands dirty and wait increasing amounts of time before washing them. The therapist helps the person cope with the anxiety that waiting produces; after the exercise has been repeated a number of times, the anxiety diminishes. People with social phobia may be encouraged to spend time in feared social situations without giving in to the temptation to flee and to make small social blunders and observe how people respond to them. Since the response is usually far less harsh than the person fears, these anxieties are lessened. People with PTSD may be supported through recalling their traumatic event in a safe situation, which helps reduce the fear it produces. CBT therapists also teach deep breathing and other types of exercises to relieve anxiety and encourage relaxation.

Exposure-based behavioral therapy has been used for many years to treat specific phobias. The person gradually encounters the object or situation that is feared, perhaps at first only through pictures or tapes, then later face-to-face. Often the therapist will accompany the person to a feared situation to provide support and guidance.

CBT is undertaken when people decide they are ready for it and with their permission and cooperation. To be effective, the therapy must be directed at the person's specific anxieties and must be tailored to his or her needs. There are no side effects other than the discomfort of temporarily increased anxiety.

CBT or behavioral therapy often lasts about twelve weeks. It may be conducted individually or with a group of people who have similar problems. Group therapy is particularly effective for social phobia. Often "homework" is assigned for participants to complete between sessions. There is some evidence that the benefits of CBT last longer than those of medication for people with panic disorder, and the same may be true for OCD, PTSD, and social phobia. If a disorder recurs at a later date, the same therapy can be used to treat it successfully a second time.

Medication can be combined with psychotherapy for specific anxiety disorders, and this is the best treatment approach for many people.

If you think you have an anxiety disorder, the first person you should see is your family or VA doctor. A physician can determine whether the symptoms that alarm you are due to an anxiety disorder, another medical condition, or both.

If an anxiety disorder is diagnosed, the next step is usually seeing a mental health professional. The practitioners who are most helpful with anxiety disorders are those who have training in CBT and/or behavioral therapy, and who are open to using medication if it is needed.

You should feel comfortable talking with the mental health professional you choose. If you do not, you should seek help elsewhere. Once you find a mental health professional with whom you are comfortable,

**TAKING MEDICATIONS**

Before taking medication for an anxiety disorder:

- Ask your doctor to tell you about the effects and side effects of the drug.
- Tell your doctor about any alternative therapies or over-the-counter medications you are using.
- Ask your doctor when and how the medication should be stopped. Some drugs can't be stopped abruptly but must be tapered off slowly under a doctor's supervision.
- Work with your doctor to determine which medication is right for you and what dosage is best.
- Be aware that some medications are effective only if they are taken regularly and that symptoms may recur if the medication is stopped.

the two of you should work as a team and make a plan to treat your anxiety disorder together.

Remember that once you start on medication, it is important not to stop taking it abruptly. Certain drugs must be tapered off under the supervision of a doctor or bad reactions can occur. Make sure you talk to the doctor who prescribed your medication before you stop taking it. If you are having trouble with side effects, it's possible that they can be eliminated by adjusting how much medication you take and when you take it.

Most insurance plans, including health maintenance organizations (HMOs), cover treatment for anxiety disorders. Check with your insurance company and find out. If you don't have insurance, the Health and Human Services division of your county government may offer mental health care at a public mental health center that charges people according to how much they are able to pay. If you are on public assistance, you may be able to get care through your state Medicaid plan.

## How Can Family and Friends Assist in the Healing Process

Many people with anxiety disorders benefit from joining a self-help or support group and sharing their problems and achievements with others. Internet chat rooms can also be useful in this regard, but any advice received over the Internet should be used with caution, as Internet acquaintances have usually never seen each other and false identities are common. Talking with a trusted friend or member of the clergy can also provide support, but it is not a substitute for care from a mental health professional.

Stress-management techniques and meditation can help people with anxiety disorders calm themselves and may enhance the effects of therapy. There is preliminary evidence that aerobic exercise may have a calming effect. Since caffeine, certain illicit drugs, and even some over-the-counter cold medications can aggravate the symptoms of anxiety disorders, they should be avoided. Check with your physician or pharmacist before taking any additional medications.

The family is very important in the recovery of a person with an anxiety disorder. Ideally, the family should be supportive but not help perpetuate their loved one's symptoms. Family members should not trivialize the disorder or demand improvement without treatment. If your family is doing either of these things, you may want to show them this chapter so they can become educated allies and help you succeed in therapy.

## Resources Available

Visit the National Library of Medicine's MedlinePlus: www.nlm.nih.gov/medlineplus

En Español: medlineplus.gov/spanish

# 7

# GRIEF

## What Is Grief?

Grief is a normal and natural reaction to loss. It is also a natural and necessary part of healing after a loss. People usually grieve when someone they love dies. But a person can also feel grief after losing something meaningful or valuable.

People are often surprised by the reactions they have when they are grieving. For example, they may be in shock when first learning of the death of a loved one. They may be angry at God, themselves, the person who died, or someone who they think is responsible for the loss or death. They may also feel guilty about not having done something differently before the person died.

Major losses and death may cause some changes in life, sometimes very significant changes. These changes may include having to parent alone, getting used to single life after divorce, or going back to work. Going through these changes may add more stress, so it's important to have support from others. It's possible to find support by talking to a psychologist, chaplain, or other spiritual advisor, or to family members, friends, a health care professional, or other helpful people.

Losses can include:

Divorce or break-up of an important relationship
Death of a loved one
Death of comrades (combat or noncombat related)
Loss of a pet
Loss of a sense of safety
Loss of meaning and purpose in life

Loss of physical health or a physical part of oneself
Loss of ability to relate or connect with others
Loss of identity
Loss of self-esteem

Common thoughts, feelings, and reactions caused by loss and grief:

Denial
Disbelief or doubt
Confusion
Shock
Sadness
Yearning or longing
Anger
Shame
Despair
Guilt
Regret
Feeling empty and/or depressed
Having a hard time relating to or connecting with others
Thinking that a part of oneself has died
Hopelessness about the future
Thinking things aren't as important as they once were
Getting tearful or crying easily
Feeling restless or irritable
Having upset stomach, headaches, or other physical pains
Existing health problems becoming worse or new physical problems appearing
Loss of appetite
Having a hard time sleeping or sleeping much more than usual
Having little energy

## How Long Does Grieving Last?

The grief period is different for everyone. A person's personality as well as family, cultural, spiritual, and religious beliefs and practices can influence how one responds to loss. It can take many months for the painful feelings and thoughts to go away. Grief has its own timeline. But, over time, grief will begin to decrease. A grieving person will likely have good days and bad days. And it's normal and expected that the grief might return "out of the blue"; that's part of the grief process. Important dates, like anniversaries or birthdays, can bring back intense feelings of grief.

Grieving usually involves feeling sadness and other feelings related to the loss. It often involves talking about the loss with other people. However, sometimes people have a hard time grieving because:

They don't deal with their grief because it's uncomfortable.
They were raised to believe that they should never be sad and were told that, "crying is for babies."
They believe that feelings are a sign of weakness, or that grieving is only OK at funerals.
Friends and family tell them, "You have to stay strong and move on with your life."

These are mistaken beliefs that get in the way of letting the grieving process happen naturally, and may result in even worse grief from which it's then harder to recover.

## Warning Signs

There are several warning signs that may suggest that a person is having a severe grief reaction and needs help coping. Ignoring the warning signs may make the grief last longer and/or make the grieving more difficult. There are professionals and groups with expertise that can help. It is strongly recommended that a professional provider be contacted *immediately* if any of the following conditions or warning signs are present:

Thinking about or planning to commit suicide or engage in self-harm
After several days, the grief reaction getting in the way of self-care, such as eating and taking a shower
Finding distractions to avoid grieving, such as:
Not *talking* about the loss
Not being honest about the *thoughts and feelings* that are occurring since the loss
Not talking or thinking about *memories* related to the loss
Unable to function for weeks to months after the loss
Unable to carry out work, school, or family responsibilities

## Coping with Grief

It is hard to accept and work through grief, but not dealing with it can lead to depression. Coping with loss and grief in healthy ways can prevent problems from getting worse. Here are some things that can help the grieving process happen naturally, which will help avoid depression:

People can be hard on themselves following a loss. In fact, *it's okay to grieve*. It takes courage to grieve following the loss of someone important.

Be patient. Take time to grieve. It may not feel like it at first, but with time the pain will ease and it will be easier to get on with normal activities.

Join a support group where personal stories can be shared with others. It is often helpful to spend time with people who have gone through a similar loss.

Seek helpful people, such as family or friends, or a chaplain or other spiritual advisor.

Seek out professional consultation with a psychologist or social worker or other health care professional if the grieving persists.

Even though it can be hard to ask for help, it's important to know that no one has to experience grief alone. It's easy to feel alone and to think that no one else could possibly be going through the same thing. However, often other people *are* going through the same thing, or have had a similar experience coping with a loss, and they may be having the same thoughts and dealing with the same issues.

Talking about feelings, although uncomfortable, is an important step to getting past grief. Mental health care professionals can offer a private, safe place to talk about grief and assist with the grieving process.

## Research

Although research into the prevalence and intensity of grief symptoms in war veterans is limited, clinicians recognize the importance for veterans of grieving the loss of comrades. Grief symptoms can include sadness; longing; missing the deceased; nonacceptance of the death; feeling the death was unfair; anger; feeling stunned, dazed, or shocked; emptiness; preoccupation with thoughts and images of the deceased; loss of enjoyment; difficulties in trusting others; social impairments; and guilt concerning the circumstances of the death. Recent research results, although limited to one sample of Vietnam combat veterans in a residential rehabilitation unit for posttraumatic stress disorder (PTSD), have supported findings in the general bereavement literature that unresolved grief can be detected as a distress syndrome distinct from depression and anxiety. In this sample of combat veterans, grief symptoms were detected at very high levels of intensity, thirty years postloss. The intensity of symptoms experienced after thirty years was similar to that reported in community samples of grieving spouses and parents at six months postloss. This supports clinical observations that unresolved grief, if left untreated, can continue unabated and increases the distress load of veterans. The existence of a distinct and intense set of grief symptoms indicates the need for clinical attention to grief in the treatment plan.

## Attachment and Bonding Are Essential to Unit Cohesiveness

Bonds with unit members are described by many veterans as some of the closest relationships they have formed in their lives. During Vietnam, soldiers were rotated in and out of units on individual schedules. Nevertheless, the percentage of returning veterans with PTSD who also report bereavement-related distress is high. In the Iraq conflict, young service personnel and reservists have remained with their units throughout training and deployment. Levels of mutual trust and respect, unit cohesiveness, and affective bonding have been further strengthened by the experiences of deployment. While bonding and attachment to the unit may result in some protection against subsequent development of PTSD, unresolved bereavement may be expected to be associated with increased distress over the lifespan unless these losses are acknowledged and grief symptoms treated on a timely basis.

## Traumatic Grief

Traumatic grief refers to the experience of the *sudden loss* of a significant and close attachment. Having a close buddy, identification with service personnel in the unit, and experiencing multiple losses were the strongest predictors of grief symptoms in the above sample of Vietnam veterans. Other factors that may influence the development of prolonged grief syndrome include: survivor guilt; feelings of powerlessness in not being able to prevent the death; anger at others who are thought to have caused the death; anger at oneself for committing a self-perceived error resulting in the death; tasks of survival in combat taking precedence over grieving; not being able to show emotional vulnerability; numbing and defending against overwhelming emotions; not having an opportunity in the field to acknowledge the death; and increased sense of vulnerability by seeing someone close killed. Factors important in the Iraq War may include exposure to significant numbers of civilian casualties, exposure to death from friendly fire or accidents resulting from massive and rapid troop movements, and concern about culpability for having caused death or harm to civilians in cities. These factors may contribute to experiences of shock, disbelief, and self-blame that increase risk of traumatic and complicated grief reactions.

### *Experiences That Can Influence the Development of Intense Grief: What We Learned from Vietnam*

The sudden loss of attachments takes many forms in the war zone. Service personnel may experience overwhelming self-blame for events that are not under their control, including deaths during the chaos of firefights, accidents and failures of equipment, medical triage, and casualties from friendly fire. The everyday infantryman from Vietnam lived his mistakes over and over again, perhaps in order to find some way of relieving pain and guilt from the death of friends. Many medics during Vietnam suffered tremendously when they were not able to save members of their unit, especially when they identified strongly with the men under their care. Pilots called in to fire close to troops were overcome with guilt when their ordinance hit American service personnel even while saving a majority of men. Officers felt unique responsibility for the subordinates under their care and suffered undue guilt and grief when results of combat were damaging. Those who worked closely with civilians were often shocked when they witnessed deaths of people with whom they had come to develop mutual trust. Deaths of civilian women and children were difficult to bear.

Many of these same experiences can be expected to affect combat troops in Iraq.

## Normal vs. Pathological Grief

Bereavement is a universal experience. Intense emotions, including sadness, longing, anger, and guilt, are reactions to the loss of a close person. Common in the first days and weeks of grieving are intense emotions, usually experienced as coming in waves lasting twenty minutes to an hour, with accompanying somatic sensations in the stomach, tightness in the throat, shortness of breath, intense fatigue, feeling faint, agitation, and helplessness. Lack of motivation, loss of interest in outside activities, and social withdrawal are also fairly common. A person experiencing normal grief will have a gradual decline in symptoms and distress. When grief symptoms remain at severely discomforting levels, even after two months, a referral to a clinician can be considered. If intense symptoms persist after six months, a diagnosis of complicated grief can be made and there is a definite indication for clinical intervention. Complicated grief prolonged over time has been shown to have negative effects on health, social functioning, and mental health.

## Acute Traumatic Grief

Survivors of traumatic events can experience acute symptoms of distress including intense agitation, self-accusations, high-risk behaviors, suicidal ideation, and intense outbursts of anger, superimposed on the symptoms of normal bereavement. Service personnel who lose their comrades in battle have been known to make heroic efforts to save them or recover their bodies. Some have reacted with rage at the enemy, risking their lives with little thought ("gone berserk" or "kill crazy"). Some withdraw and become loners, seldom or never again making friends; some express extreme anger at the events and personnel that brought them to the conflict. Some are inclined to mask their emotions. Any sign of vulnerability or "losing" it can indicate that they are not tough enough to handle combat. Delaying grief may well postpone problems that can become chronic symptoms weeks, months, and years later. The returning veteran who has developed PTSD and/or depression may well be masking his or her grief symptoms.

### *Assessment and Treatment of Acute Grief in Returning Veterans*

Clinical judgment is necessary in deciding when and how to treat acute grief reactions, especially when they are accompanied by a diagnosis of acute stress disorder (ASD). While a cognitive-behavioral treatment package that includes exposure therapy has been shown to prevent the development of PTSD some persons with ASD, exposure therapy during the initial stages of grief may often be contraindicated, because it may place great emotional strain on someone only just bereaved. Bereavement researchers also are hesitant to treat grief in the first few months of a normal loss, wishing not to interfere with a natural healing process. In the early stages of grief, symptoms may be experienced as intense, but this is normal for the first days, weeks, and months. Those surviving a traumatic loss in the war zone will be more likely to mask intense feelings of sadness, pain, vulnerability, anxiety, anger, and guilt. Balancing other traumatic experiences with the intensity of grief may feel overwhelming. Therefore it is important to assess and respect the individual soldier's ability to cope and manage these feelings at any time. A soldier may be relieved to know that someone understands how he or she feels after losing a buddy, or experiencing other losses including civilians or multiple deaths in the field, and communication with a clinician may be a first step in coming to terms with loss. However, that soldier may not be ready to probe more deeply into feelings and circumstances. Care and patience in the assessment process, as well as in beginning treatment, is essential.

Treatment during the acute stages of grief would best include acknowledgement of the loss, communication of understanding of the depth of feelings, encouragement to recover positive memories of the deceased, recognition of the good intentions of the survivor to come to the aid of the deceased, education about what to expect during the course of acute grief, and encouragement of distraction and relaxation techniques as a temporary palliative. Efforts to reduce symptoms of PTSD and depression as comorbid disorders would take precedence over grief symptoms in the initial phases of treatment, unless the loss itself is the main cause of distress.

## Assessment of Complicated Grief in Returning Veterans

Grief symptoms including sadness, distress, guilt, anger, intrusive thoughts, and preoccupation with the death should be declining after about six months during a normal grieving process. If symptoms remain very high after six months, clinical intervention is warranted. There are several instruments that may be helpful in assessing a complicated grief. The Inventory of Complicated Grief-Revised is perhaps most widely used and reflects current bereavement research. Another instrument is the Texas Revised Inventory of Grief, which has been used in a variety of populations and has been well validated. Both allow comparisons with normative populations.

### *Treatment of Complicated Grief in Returning Veterans*

There have been no outcome studies of treatments of veterans for prolonged and complicated grief symptoms at this time. Clinical experience supports the importance of education about normal and complicated grief processes, education about the cognitive processes of guilt, restructuring of cognitive distortions of events that might lead to excessive guilt, looking at the function of anger in bereavement, restoring positive memories of the deceased, restoration and acknowledgment of caring feelings toward the deceased, affirming resilience and positive coping, retelling the story of the death, and learning to tolerate painful feelings as part of the grieving process. These activities can be provided in individual treatment or in closed groups.

Regardless of the techniques that are used, what is central to treating veterans for prolonged and complicated grief is recognition of the significance of their losses, provision of an opportunity to talk about the deceased, restructuring of distorted thoughts of guilt, and validation of the pain and intensity of their feelings. What is most essential is that bereavement and loss be treated in addition to PTSD and depression for a more complete recovery.

## Helping Bereaved Military Children

Robin F. Goodman, PhD, Judith A. Cohen, MD, and Stephen J. Cozza, MD

The joy of family reunion after a military deployment is often more than children or parents even hoped for. However, for some children the reunion never comes. Sadly, some children must cope with the death of a parent.

There are often no words to console a child or explain what happened. But surviving family members, adults, and a caring community can help grieving military children. Below are some suggestions to help ease children's pain and support their resilience after a death.

- Be honest and open. All children need information appropriate to their age. Use clear language that includes the term "death" rather than euphemisms (e.g., "loss," "gone to sleep") that may confuse children. Follow the child's lead and need for explanations of what happened. Rather than having just one conversation, stay open to ongoing questions and discussions.
- Provide a sense of safety and security. Reestablishing routines and structure go a long way toward providing children a comforting sense of stability in the midst of changes. This can be done in the simplest of ways, for example, keeping up with ongoing afterschool activities and regular bedtimes.
- Be a good detective. Pay attention to how and what your child is communicating. Children often show their feelings and thoughts by their behaviors. Take a step back, ask the right questions, listen, and validate their feelings.
- Support expression of feelings. Drawing, writing, playing, or reading books about grief can help children learn about and express feelings. Let them know all feelings are acceptable and help children find healthy ways to channel them.
- Be a good role model. Children look to caregivers for examples of how to react and cope. It's okay for grownups to show their emotions, as long as they are not out of control or frightening to children. Adult expressions of sadness can model healthy ways of dealing with difficult feelings. For example, you can say: "I'm crying because I feel sad your dad is missing your soccer game; it's okay for you to cry when you miss him too."
- Help children learn about the person and stay connected. Sharing stories, photos, and memories helps keep the person alive in the child's heart and keeps the person a part of the child's identity. For example, you can say:
  - "Even though dad died, we can still remember how much fun we had together on our beach vacations."
- Keep perspective about non-grief-related areas. Remember that children are still moving forward in their lives. Be aware of other developmental milestones and issues your children are facing at different ages, such as peer pressure or worry over school work, which may or may not relate to the person who died. Grief may make some of these times more difficult; for example, a teen not having his dad to teach him to drive.

- Partner with other trusted adults in your child's world. Educate others about your child's grief and collaborate with them to support your child. For example, give and get feedback from teachers and coaches.
- Look for peer support. Children and caregivers can benefit from being with others who "know what it's like." Some can benefit from groups that mix military and nonmilitary families, others prefer military specific groups such as those found on a base or offered by Tragedy Assistance Program for Survivors (TAPS), which holds Survivor Seminars and Good Grief Camps regionally across the country.
- Take care of yourself. The better and stronger you are, the better caregiver you will be to your children. This includes taking care of your physical health (e.g., eating, sleeping, exercising, relaxing, etc.). This can also decrease children's worry about the people they depend on. Take care of your emotional health as well by managing stress and connecting to supportive friends and family who can help you.
- Be alert to children who may be having difficulty. Some children may have a traumatic reaction. Some signs that children need more help include their being bothered by upsetting and recurring thoughts or images of the deceased person or the death, avoidance of military-related reminders or talk about the person who died, and unusual irritability or jumpiness. If you notice these behaviors in your child consider seeking professional help.
- Seek professional support. Caregivers and children may believe they should be able to handle their grief on their own or that they are weak if they need help, and neither is true. Important communities to reach out for assistance include school, community, medical, mental health, and faith-based resources when needed.

Grief is a new experience for many people. With any new experience, you can help to learn more about it, get answers to questions, and develop strategies to help you and your child get through it.

# 8

# Stigma

Many veterans, in trying to make sense of their traumatic war experiences, blame themselves or feel guilty in some way. They may feel bad about something(s) they did or didn't do in the war zone. Feelings of guilt or self-blame cause much distress and can prevent a person from reaching out for help.

Therefore, even though it is hard, it is very important to talk about guilt feelings with a counselor or doctor.

Depression and grief can get in the way of seeking help because depressed people tend to feel worn out and think that they are worthless, hopeless, and helpless. It's very common for depressed people to believe that nothing will help.

Often people have an incorrect view of what getting help means, or may be skeptical of treatment. For some, there is a stigma or shame attached to getting help, especially within the military. This type of thinking gets in the way of getting needed help. Effective treatment is available for depression. It takes courage to seek help for depression, and the earlier seeking out treatment happens, the better!

## What Is It?

Mental health problems are not a sign of weakness. The reality is that injuries, including psychological injuries, affect the strong and the brave just like everyone else. Some of the most successful officers and enlisted personnel have experienced these problems.

But stigma about mental health issues can be a huge barrier for people who need help. The stigma associated with mental health problems continues to be highly prevalent today, despite greater public awareness and improved knowledge.

Finding the solution to your problem is a sign of strength and maturity. Getting assistance from others is sometimes the only way to solve something. For example, if you cannot scale a wall on your own and need comrades to do so, you use them! Knowing when and how to get help is actually part of military training.

## The Extent of the Problem

Those in the military are often hesitant to seek help for depression because of the following thoughts.

"Getting help will affect my career."

Service members are more likely to get in trouble if they *don't* seek help, because not getting help can make problems worse. Not getting help for depression can result in negative behavior toward coworkers and poor work performance, which can cause other problems between a service member and others.

"My leaders will have access to my mental health records."

Information between a doctor and a service member *does* become part of the service member's medical record. Technically, the information is available to commanding officers upon their request. But in most cases, confidentiality is maintained between providers at a military treatment facility (MTF) and the person seeking help. Chaplains and other service providers should explain the limits of confidentiality or privacy to a service member. If they don't, just ask.

"My service records will show my mental health information."

Military service records don't contain mental health information unless the service member was officially ordered to get help or if was found unfit or unsuitable for military duty.

"My command discourages me from getting help."

There are local community resources available to service members who don't feel comfortable going through the military. Service members and their unit will benefit if they seek and receive help for their problems before they get worse and risk lives and military readiness.

## What Are Your Options?

Tune into negative thinking and examine thoughts for thinking errors.

Avoid the urge to be alone. Be with other people. Confide in someone—it's healthier than self-isolating.

Know that a low mood can improve, even if not right away. Feeling better takes time and patience.

Set small goals despite feeling depressed. Have a friend, family member, or mental health professional see if goals are realistic and reachable.

Put off very important decisions or changes until the depression has lifted. Before deciding to make major changes such as changing jobs or getting married or divorced, discuss it with others who have a more neutral view of the situation.

Be around positive and supportive people.

Don't use alcohol or drugs (unless the drugs are prescribed and taken as directed). Alcohol and/or drug use can increase depression in the long run.

Many people believe that they don't deserve to feel better or that they won't ever get better. Don't buy into these thoughts. They are just negative thoughts and they aren't true! Everyone has the power and ability to change negative thinking. *Everyone deserves to get better and they will if they keep working at it.*

## How Family and Friends Can Assist

The benefits to individuals and families of tackling stigma include a reversal of the negative effects of discrimination listed above. Families and friends must be loving and supportive—and firm, to ensure the individual continues to receive medication and takes all prescribed medicines.

All of us, especially medical professionals, need to consider our own attitudes and awareness. The recognition that anyone will break down if stress is high enough should help free us from an "us and them" attitude.

For mental health practitioners, enabling service users to influence service development is another strong antistigma move. Collaboration with stigmatized people on projects has had major impacts on attitudes in other arenas of discrimination. Antidiscrimination work may mean writing an appropriate reference for someone who has had treatment, or supporting a service user through an industrial tribunal. A cognitive-behavior-therapy approach can help individuals to overcome felt stigma and cope better with discrimination, but we should avoid giving the impression that the stigma is their fault.

## Resources Available

No one should have to deal with grief or depression alone or the perceived stigma associated with it. It can be hard to ask for help but healthcare professionals can provide a safe place to talk about feelings and help with the healing process. Here are a few resources:

*An installation's support services can provide information and support.* Support services include a chaplain, a MTF, and family advocacy programs and family centers. Phone numbers can be found in the installation's military directory.

*Talk to command.* Check in with a leader about how to handle a stressful situation before the situation gets out of control. Keeping leadership informed is good practice.

*Make an appointment with a primary-care provider (PCP).* Ask the PCP about available treatment options, and a referral to a mental health practitioner if that is indicated.

*Military OneSource.* Military OneSource provides brief counseling to active duty military personnel and their families, including Reservists and the National Guard: (1-800-342-9647); www.militaryonesource.com.

*The Tragedy Assistance Program for Survivors (TAPS)* is a nonprofit veterans service organization that has a wide range of free services to all those affected by the death of a loved one in the armed forces: 1-800-959-TAPS (1-800-959-8277) or www.TAPS.org.

*Vet centers* offer readjustment counseling for veterans and their families. Vet center staff is available toll free at 1-800-905-4675 (Eastern) and 1-866-496-8838 (Pacific); www.vetcenter.va.gov.

*Veteran Affairs Resources.* VA medical centers and vet centers provide veterans with affordable mental health services. Health insurance companies cover costs, or services cost little or nothing, according to a veteran's ability to pay. The VA medical center system's specialized posttraumatic stress disorder (PTSD) clinics and programs can provide educational information and diagnostic evaluations concerning PTSD to eligible veterans. Following deployment to a combat zone after discharge, veterans who have enrolled for VA services are qualified for two years of care for conditions potentially related to their service. See: www.va.gov.

*Local community services* can include crisis centers, mental health centers, or suicide prevention centers.

*Find mental health providers locally.* See: therapists.psychologytoday.com/ppc/prof_search.php.

*Suicide hotlines.* The national suicide prevention lifeline is available twenty-four hours. 1-800-273-TALK (1-800-273-8255) or 1-800-SUICIDE (1-800-784-2433). Both suicide hotlines will connect the caller to a certified crisis center nearest to the location from where the call is placed. See: www.suicidepreventionlifeline.org.

# 9

# ALCOHOL / DRUGS

Dependence on alcohol and drugs is our most serious national public-health problem. It is prevalent among rich and poor, in all regions of the country, and all ethnic and social groups.

Millions of Americans misuse or are dependent on alcohol or drugs. Most of them have families who suffer the consequences, often serious, of living with this illness. If there is alcohol or drug dependence in your family, remember you are not alone.

## The Extent of the Problem

It's common for troops to "self-medicate." They drink or abuse drugs to numb out the difficult thoughts, feelings, and memories related to war-zone experiences. While alcohol or drugs may seem to offer a quick solution, they actually lead to more problems. At the same time, a vast majority of people in our society drink. Sometimes it can be difficult to know if your drinking is actually a problem.

Most individuals who abuse alcohol or drugs have jobs and are productive members of society, creating a false hope in the family that "it's not that bad."

The problem is that addiction tends to worsen over time, hurting both the addicted person and all the family members. It is especially damaging to young children and adolescents.

People with this illness really may believe that they drink normally or that "everyone" takes drugs. These false beliefs are called denial; this denial is a part of the illness.

Drug- or alcohol-dependence disorders are medical conditions that can be effectively treated. Millions of Americans and their families are in healthy recovery from this disease.

If someone close to you misuses alcohol or drugs, the first step is to be honest about the problem and to seek help for yourself, your family, and your loved one.

Treatment can occur in a variety of settings, in many different forms, and for different lengths of time. Stopping the alcohol or drug use is the first step to recovery, and most people need help to stop. Often a person with alcohol or drug dependence will need treatment provided by professionals just as with other diseases. Your doctor may be able to guide you.

Many military personnel experience stress related to their deployment, service, and return home.

These quite natural stress reactions can range from mild to severe and may be either short-lived or persist for a very long time. One common approach to managing stress that seems a simple and easy solution is use of alcohol or drugs. Military personnel, like civilians, may use alcohol and drugs as a way to relax or reduce anxiety and other bad feelings. In some cases, alcohol and drugs are not only used to decrease stress but also to manage severe symptoms that can arise from a traumatic experience in the war zone. You might find yourself drinking or using drugs for a variety of reasons when under stress or after trauma, including to:

- Help yourself sleep
- Decrease sadness
- Relax
- Help yourself be around others
- Decrease emotional pain
- Increase pleasurable experience
- "Drown" your worries
- Keep upsetting memories from coming to mind
- Escape present difficulties
- "Shake off" stress
- Calm anxiety

## Substance Abuse and the Military

Substance abuse is a growing problem in the military because of the tremendous strains both on military personnel themselves and their families

Some have experienced devastating consequences, including family disintegration, mental health disorders, and even suicide. Research conducted by RAND has shown that 25 to 30 percent of Iraq and Afghanistan war veterans have reported symptoms of a mental disorder or cognitive impairment. Post-traumatic stress disorder (PTSD) is the most common, and traumatic brain injury may be a causal factor in some reported symptoms. Although less common, substance use is also a large concern, with aggregated data from the Substance Abuse and Mental Health Services Administration's annual household survey revealing that from 2004 to 2006, 7.1 percent of veterans (an estimated 1.8 million persons 18 or older) met criteria for a past-year substance use disorder.

Problems with alcohol and nicotine abuse are the most prevalent and pose a significant risk to the health of veterans as well as to Reserve component and National Guard soldiers. At greatest risk are deployed personnel with combat exposures, as they are more apt to engage in new-onset heavy weekly drinking, binge drinking, and to suffer alcohol-related problems; as well as smoking initiation and relapse. Within this group, Reserve and National Guard personnel and younger service members are particularly vulnerable to subsequent drinking problems. And although alcohol problems are frequently reported among veterans, few are referred to alcohol treatment.

The military today have a number of things working against them, causing them to return home addicted to drugs or alcohol or suffering from mental illness. The military today regularly prescribes medication to help ease stress and anxiety, to help with physical pain, or to keep them alert when they need to be. These kinds of prescription drugs, while they might be necessary in a war situation, become addicting and on their return to normal life, they can't do without them. Many other members of the military are self-medicating and becoming addicted in the process.

To gain a fuller understanding of these burgeoning issues, the Millennium Cohort Study—the largest prospective study in military history—is following a representative sample of U.S. military personnel from 2001 to 2022. Early findings highlight the importance of prevention in this group, given the long-term effects of combat-related problems and the ensuing difficulties experienced in seeking or being referred to treatment, likely because of stigma and other real and perceived barriers. To fill this need, a host of government agencies, researchers, public health entities and others are working together to adapt and test proven prevention interventions, as well as drug abuse treatments, for potential use with military and veteran populations and their families.

To address the social problems both caused by and contributing to drug use, the Department of Defense and partners are developing and testing novel treatment approaches with veterans. For example, Rosen's Money Management Intervention trains those in drug treatment to better manage their money by linking access to funds to treatment goal completion. For relapse prevention, McKay's telephone treatment approach delivers counseling at home for several months once a veteran has completed an initial face-to-face treatment episode.

While NIDA is striving to expand its portfolio of research related to trauma, stress, and substance use and abuse among veterans and their families, a number of promising projects are already being funded. These include studies on: smoking cessation and PTSD, behavioral interventions for the dually diagnosed, substance use and HIV progression, and virtual reality treatment of PTSD and substance abuse. Additionally, NIDA's National Drug Abuse Treatment Clinical Trials Network (CTN) is developing, in conjunction with researchers from the Veterans Administration, a protocol concept on the treatment of PTSD / SUD in veteran populations.

Further, efforts are under way to make it easier for veterans to access treatments. Research on drug courts, for example, is now being applied to developing courts for veterans, the former having demonstrated their effectiveness in addressing nonviolent crimes by drug abusers and ushering them into needed treatment instead of prison. Because the criminal justice system is a frequent treatment referral source for veterans, such specialized courts may give them the opportunity to access the services and support they may not otherwise receive. While New York has the only court that exclusively handles nonviolent crimes committed by veterans, other states are considering establishing such courts.

## How Does It Manifest Itself?

### *Warning Signs*

Not all drinking is harmful and moderate drinking might even be good for you. However, at-risk or heavy drinkers can face serious risks unless they take action.

*Injuries.* Drinking too much increases your chances of being injured or even killed. Alcohol is a factor, for example, in about 60 percent of fatal burn injuries, drowning, and homicides; 50 percent of severe trauma injuries and sexual assaults; and 40 percent of fatal motor vehicle crashes, suicides, and fatal falls.

*Health problems.* Heavy drinkers have a greater risk of liver disease, heart disease, sleep disorders, depression, stroke, bleeding from the stomach, sexually transmitted infections from unsafe sex, and several types of cancer. They may also have problems managing diabetes, high blood pressure, and other conditions.

*Birth defects.* Drinking during pregnancy can cause brain damage and other serious problems in the baby. Because it is not yet known whether any amount of alcohol is safe for a developing baby, women who are pregnant or may become pregnant should not drink.

*Alcohol-use disorders.* Generally known as alcoholism and alcohol abuse, alcohol use disorders are medical conditions that doctors can diagnose when a patient's drinking causes distress or harm. In the United States, about eighteen million people have an alcohol-use disorder.

See if you recognize any of these symptoms in yourself or a loved one:

In the past year, have you had times when you ended up drinking more, or longer, than you intended?

More than once wanted to cut down or stop drinking, or tried to, but couldn't?

More than once gotten into situations while or after drinking that increased your chances of getting hurt (such as driving, swimming, using machinery, walking in a dangerous area, or having unsafe sex)?

Had to drink much more than you once did to get the effect you want? Or found that your usual number of drinks had much less effect than before?

Continued to drink even though it was making you feel depressed or anxious or adding to another health problem? Or after having had a memory blackout?

Spent a lot of time drinking? Or being sick or getting over other aftereffects?

Continued to drink even though it was causing trouble with your family or friends?

Found that drinking—or being sick from drinking—often interfered with taking care of your home or family? Or caused job troubles?

Given up or cut back on activities that were important or interesting to you, or gave you pleasure, in order to drink?

More than once gotten arrested, been held at a police station, or had other legal problems because of your drinking?

Found that when the effects of alcohol were wearing off, you had withdrawal symptoms, such as trouble sleeping, shakiness, restlessness, nausea, sweating, a racing heart, or a seizure? Or sensed things that were not there?

If you or a loved one have any symptoms, then alcohol may already be a cause for concern. The more symptoms you have, the more urgent the need for change. A health professional can look at the number, pattern, and severity of symptoms to see whether an alcohol use disorder is present and help you decide the best course of action.

Alcoholism is chronic alcohol abuse that results in a physical dependence on alcohol and an inability to stop or limit drinking.

Warning signs of an alcohol problem include:

- Frequent excessive drinking
- Having thoughts that you should cut down
- Feeling guilty or bad about your drinking

- Others becoming annoyed with you or criticizing how much you drink
- Drinking in the morning to calm your nerves
- Problems with work, family, school, or other regular activities caused by drinking

Initially, alcohol and drugs may seem to make things better. They may help you sleep, forget problems, or feel more relaxed. But any short-term benefit can turn sour fast. In the long run, using alcohol and drugs to cope with stress causes a whole new set of very serious problems, and worsens the original problems that lead you to drink or use. Alcohol and drug abuse can cause problems with your family life, health, mental well-being, relationships, finances, employment, spirituality, and sense of self-worth.

Think about family impact as an example. It's difficult to create good relationships when you are regularly drunk or high. Being intoxicated decreases intimacy and creates an inability to communicate well. Family members can feel rejected by someone who is always under the influence. In addition, witnessing someone's behavior while under the influence can be distressing. Children may not understand the aggressive behavior, the shutting down, or the hiding out that can occur along with substance use. The fallout from an accident or an arrest can have a long-lasting impact on a family. Alcohol and drug problems are dangerous for loved ones, because they are often linked with family violence and driving while intoxicated.

### *When is Use of Alcohol a Problem?*

It is often hard to decide whether alcohol or drug use is becoming a problem. It can happen gradually, and sometimes can be hard to notice by the person who is using. Here are things that people sometimes say to themselves to convince themselves that they do not have a problem. Do you recognize any?

- "I just drink beer (wine)."
- "I don't drink every day."
- "I don't use hard drugs."
- "I've never missed a day of work."
- "I'm not an alcoholic."
- "I don't need help, I can handle it."
- "I gave it up for three weeks last year myself."

Alcohol or drug use can be considered a problem when it causes difficulties, even in minor ways.

Here are some questions that you can ask yourself to see if you are developing a problem:

*Have friends or family members commented on how much or how often you drink?*
*Have you have found yourself feeling guilty about your drinking or drug use?*
*Have you found yourself drinking (using) more over time?*
*Have you tried to cut down your alcohol (drug) use?*
*Does your drinking (using drugs) ever affect your ability to fulfill personal obligations such as parenting or work?*
*Do you drink (use) in situations that are physically dangerous such as driving or operating machinery while under the influence?*
*Have you found that you need more alcohol (drug) to get the same effect?*

If you find that you are answering "yes" to one or more of these questions, perhaps it is time to reevaluate your use, cut back, and seek help from friends, family, or a professional.

## What Are the Treatment Options?

If you think that alcohol (drug) use has become (or is becoming) a problem for you, there are a number of things that you can do. First, recognize that you are not alone and that others are available to lend support. Second, find help. Getting help is the most useful tool in decreasing or stopping problem drinking or drug use, even if you have doubts about being able to quit or if you are feeling guilt about the problem. Call your health provider, contact a physician or therapist, call your local US Department of Veterns Affairs (VA) hospital, or contact your local Alcoholic's Anonymous for guidance in your recovery.

CAGE is an acronym for the following questions:

C — Have you ever felt that you should **C**UT down on your drinking?
A — Have people **A**NNOYED you by criticizing your drinking?
G — Have you ever felt bad or **G**UILTY about your drinking?
E — Have you ever had a drink first thing in the morning to steady your nerves or get rid of a hangover (i.e., as an **E**YE-OPENER)?

Individuals endorsing either three or four of the CAGE questions over the past year are most likely alcohol dependent. If the individual endorses one or two of the CAGE questions they may have current alcohol abuse. Combining the introductory screening comments with the quantity-frequency and CAGE questions can reliably predict 70 to 80 percent of individuals with alcohol abuse or dependence (Friedman et al. 2001).

The same screening tool can be adapted for illicit drug use. For example, the initial questions about the person's response to notification of deployment might uncover the use of marijuana. The health care provider can then ask quantity-frequency questions followed by the adapted CAGE.

### *Case Studies*

The following case examples describe veterans who were treated at military and VA medical facilities. Information has been modified to protect patient identities.

#### CASE 1

Specialist LR is a twenty-five-year-old single African American man who is an activated National Guardsman with four years of reserve service. He is a full-time college student and competitive athlete raised by a single mother in public housing. He has a history of minor assaults in school and his neighborhood and of exposure to street violence.

Initially trained in transportation, he was called to active duty and retrained as a military policeman to serve with his unit in Baghdad. He described enjoying the high intensity of his deployment and had become recognized by others as an informal leader because of his aggressiveness and self-confidence. He describes numerous exposures while performing convoy escort and security details. He reports coming under small arms fire on several occasions, witnessing dead and injured civilians and Iraqi soldiers and on occasion feeling powerless when forced to detour or take evasive action. He began to develop increasing mistrust of the operational environment, as the situation "on the street" seemed to deteriorate. He often felt that he and his fellow service personnel were placed in harm's way needlessly.

On a routine convoy mission, serving as driver for the lead HMMWV (HUMVEE), his vehicle was struck by an improvised explosive device (IED), showering him with shrapnel in his neck, arm, and leg. Another member of his vehicle was even more seriously injured. He described "kicking into autopilot," driving his vehicle to a safe location, and jumping out to do a battle damage assessment. He denied feeling much pain at that time. He was evacuated to the Combat Support Hospital (CSH) where he was treated and returned to duty (RTD) after several days despite requiring crutches and suffering chronic pain from retained shrapnel in his neck. He began to become angry at his command and doctors for keeping him in theater while he was unable to perform his duties effectively. He began to develop insomnia, hypervigilance, and a startle response. His initial dreams of the event became more intense and frequent and he suffered intrusive thoughts and flashbacks of the attack. He began to withdraw from his friends and suffered anhedonia, feeling detached from others, and he feared his future would be cut short. He was referred to a psychiatrist at the CSH who initiated supportive therapy and a selective serotonin reuptake inhibitor (SSRI).

After two months of unsuccessful rehabilitation for his battle injuries and worsening depressive and anxiety symptoms, he was evacuated to a stateside military medical center via a European medical center. He was screened for psychiatric symptoms and was referred for outpatient evaluation and management. He met *DSM-IV* criteria for acute PTSD and was offered medication management, supportive therapy, and group therapy, which he declined. He was treated with sertraline, trazodone, and clonazepam targeting his symptoms of insomnia, anxiety, and hyperarousal. Due to continued autonomic arousal, quetiapine was substituted for the trazodone and clonazepam for sleep and anxiety, and clonidine was started for autonomic symptoms. He responded favorably to this combination of medications. He avoided alcohol as he learned it would exacerbate symptoms. He was ambivalent about taking passes or convalescent leave to his home because of fears of being "different, irritated, or aggressive" around his family and girlfriend. After three months at the military medical center, he was sent to his demobilization site to await deactivation to his National Guard unit. He was referred to his local VA hospital to receive follow-up care.

## CASE 2

PV2 RJ is a twenty-six-year-old white female with less than twelve months of active duty service who was deployed to Iraq in September 2003. She reported excelling in high school but moved out of her house after becoming pregnant during her senior year. After graduating from high school on schedule, she worked at several jobs until she was able to become an x-ray assistant. She had been on her first duty assignment as an x-ray technician in Germany. As a single parent she attempted to make plans for her dependent five-year-old son. However, when notified of her impending deployment she needed to make hurried and unexpected care plans for her son.

Within a week of being deployed to Iraq the service member began experiencing depressed mood, decreased interest in activities, increased appetite, irritability, increased social isolation with passive suicidal ideations, and insomnia due to nightmares of the devil coming after her. She also began believing Saddam Hussein was the "Antichrist." In addition, she began experiencing command-directed auditory hallucination of the devil whispering to her that people in her unit were saying she was stupid and that she should make them shut up. At one time, the devil told her to throw things at them. Her guilt intensified as her wish to act on the voices increased. She also described seeing visual hallucinations of "monsters" that were making fun of her.

These symptoms intensified when she went from an in-processing point to her assignment in Iraq. They also worsened when she ruminated about the stresses of being in Iraq (bombs exploding, missing her son and family, disgust at other women who were seeking the attention of men). Of most concern, she was worried that she might not survive the deployment. When she was around people, she experienced palpitations, increased swearing, shaking, shortness of breath, abdominal cramping, and dizziness. In hopes of getting rid of her symptoms especially the voices and monsters, she ingested Tylenol #3s she had obtained for a minor medical procedure. After confiding her symptoms to a military friend, RJ was referred for an evaluation and was evacuated out of Iraq to the contiguous United States (CONUS) via Germany.

When she returned to CONUS, RJ also shared with the treatment team that in the week prior to deployment she believed she was drugged by a date and that he sexually assaulted her. RJ was hesitant to discuss the few memories she had of the incident, due to embarrassment. She denied any other previous traumatic events but she stated she distrusted men in general, as many men in her life had been unreliable or irresponsible. She admitted to occasional alcohol use but denied any drug use. Throughout the hospitalization, her greatest concern was being reunited with her son and leaving the military. She was treated with a combination of antidepressant and antipsychotic medications that resulted in improvement in her symptoms. Despite improvement, RJ underwent a Medical Evaluation Board for diagnoses of major depression with psychotic features and PTSD.

## CASE 3

SFC W is a forty-five-year-old divorced Operation Iraqi Freedom (OIF) Reservist who was involved in a motor vehicle accident in Afghanistan in June 2003. SFC W suffered a lumbar burst fracture and had multiple surgical procedures with instrumentation and fusion at a European military medical center, which was complicated by a deep vein thrombosis.

SFC W was transferred through the aeromedical evacuation system to a stateside medical center where he was admitted as a nonbattle injury for inpatient rehabilitation for spinal cord injury. SFC W's treatment plan consisted of a rehabilitation program involving physical and occupational therapy with goals of independent ambulation with an assistive device and to establish a bowel and bladder program. The Coumadin Clinic treated his deep vein thrombosis and he was evaluated by the traumatic brain injury program staff. Pain was controlled with MS Contin 15 mg two times a day with Oxycodone IR 5 mg one to two tabs every four to six hours as needed for breakthrough pain and Ambien 10 mg per day as needed for sleep problems. Other staff included in his care were nursing, social work, chaplain, reserve liaison, Medical Holding Company, and Medical Board staff.

SFC W was followed by the preventive medicine psychiatry service (PMPS) in accordance with the service's OIF Protocol. PMPS staff initially recommended beginning therapy with an SSRI such as Sertraline at a starting dose of 25 mgm a day to address concerning symptoms, such as his increased startle response, emotional lability, and intrusive thoughts, which the staff thought could be prodromal for an acute stress disorder (ASD). PMPS staff also incorporated a combination of hypnotic and relaxation techniques to assist SFC W with sleep and pain-related problems. Staff recommended increasing sertraline to 50 mgm per day because he reported that he was continuing to be troubled by some memories of his accident. Aside from the target symptoms that were addressed above, no other psychiatric issues were identified.

An initial postdeployment health assessment tool (PDHAT) was completed during SFC W's hospital admission. He endorsed depressive symptoms at a level of 11 (a score of 10 or above indicates a potential concern) and endorsed symptoms consistent with PTSD (one intrusive symptom, two arousal symptoms and three avoidance symptoms) at the level of a little bit.

In June 2003, SFC W was transferred to the Spinal Chord Rehabilitation Program at a VA hospital. He was able to ambulate with the assistance of a walker, pain in his back and left leg was controlled with pain medicine, and his problems with a neurogenic bowel and bladder were well controlled with a daily bowel and bladder program. Additional traumatic brain testing and Coumadin regulation was requested.

Service personnel are contacted either telephonically or at the time of a follow-up visit to the Walter Reed Army Medical Center (WRAMC) and are assessed for PTSD, depression, alcohol usage, somatic complaints, days of poor physical and/or mental health and lost productivity, and satisfaction with health care.

SFC W could not be reached by phone until the six-month PDHAT follow-up. At that time he met criteria for major depression and had symptoms consistent with criteria for PTSD at the moderate level. He reported that he had lost twenty days of productivity due to physical and mental health problems. In addition, he reported problems with pain, sleep, sexual functioning, and the fact that he will never be the same again. He is able to ambulate with the assistance of a walker within his home and uses a wheel chair for outside excursions. He continues with a bowel program. His need to self-catheterize limits his visits outside the home. He is clinically followed at a local VA by psychiatry, neurology, spinal cord program, and physical therapy. He reported taking between twenty-five to thirty-five pills a day, including Trazadone for sleep and sertraline 100 mg po BID for treatment of depression and PTSD. He has accepted his functional limitations and is trying to adapt to the changes in his lifestyle. His support system is fairly good, he has a very supportive wife, his Reserve Unit is in contact with him, and he has attended social functions in recognition of returning Reservists. A request for case management services was submitted to the VA hospital to assist SFC W in understanding his medications, adapting to his functional limitations, and understanding his long-term prognosis because of his spinal cord injury, and working through his PTSD symptoms to include trauma bereavement. Legal Assistance at WRAMC also assisted him with a claim for personal property lost as a result of his deployment to Iraq.

Prior to his deployment to Iraq, SFC W worked as a truck driver for a transportation company, a job that he will not be able to return to. His Medical Board is being processed and he will then be eligible for both Army medical retirement and veterans benefits.

## CASE 4

SGT P is a twenty-four-year-old married AD USA E5 who sustained penetrating wounds to his left arm, left ribs, and left leg in an IED attack while in Iraq. Initially his wounds were treated in Kuwait and he was MEDEVAC to a European military medical center where he underwent surgery to repair a fractured left ulna bone in the summer of 2003.

SGT P was air evacuated and admitted to the general surgery service at a state side medical center. His recovery was uncomplicated and consisted of mostly rehabilitation and wound care.

He was initially followed by general surgery, vascular surgery, and orthopedics and was then discharged to inpatient physical medicine and rehabilitation (PMR) service. While on the PMR service, he progressed to ambulating hospital distances using a Lofstrand crutch and was moderately independent with Activity of Daily Living. His pain was well controlled and he was discharged on Percocet one to two tabs every four to six hours, Motrin Tabs 600 mgm three times per day as needed, and Ambien 10 mgm every night for sleep.

SGT P was followed by the PMPS in accordance with its OIF Protocol. The PMPS staff initially met with him and offered support to set the milieu to establish a therapeutic alliance with him. His initial request was for assistance with contacting his command as he had not communicated with them since his injury and felt cut-off from his unit. During his first week in the hospital, Ambien 10 mgm po at bedtime was ordered to assist with sleep problems. He subsequently reported that Ambien was only minimally helping with his sleep problems and he was now experiencing nighttime "sweats." He denied experiencing any other arousal or intrusive symptoms and only endorsed limited avoidance of television news on OIF activities. PMPS staff discussed possible risks and benefits of starting Propranol 20 mgm nightly to limit sympathetic discharge activity. SGT P agreed and was started on Propranol 20 mgm at bedtime. Follow-up reports indicated that he was sleeping well and his autonomic hyperactivity had decreased. The use of pharmacotherapy interventions decreased his sleep disturbances and to be more open and responsive to psychotherapeutic interventions. PMPS staff also incorporated a combination of hypnotic and relaxation techniques to assist him with sleep and pain related problems. Cognitive behavioral therapy (CBT) helped him understand how his traumatic experience may have altered his thoughts and interpretations of events and what effect the altered perceptions had on his emotions and behaviors. PMPS staff also assisted him in working through feelings of anger and reinforcing his coping strategies, identifying his strengths and assets.

The initial PDHAT was completed during SGT P's inpatient admission, approximately sixteen days after his injury. At that time, he endorsed criteria for major depression and endorsed symptoms consistent with PTSD at the moderate level.

Two months after admission, SGT P was discharged from the hospital and placed on convalescent leave. He had follow-up appointments in the orthopedic and vascular clinics, physical therapy, and preventive medical psychiatry. He stayed at base hotel for the duration of his outpatient therapy.

PMPS staff followed SGT P on a regular basis during the course of the hospitalization and outpatient treatment, with visits ranging from one to three times per month. A combination of psychotherapy, hypnotherapy, and CBT interventions was provided. Ambien and Propranol were not needed after the initial discharge medications were issued. He was able to regain control over the intrusive and arousal symptoms that he had been experiencing as a result of his deployment experience. Psychotherapeutic interventions assisted him in understanding the effect that his thoughts were having on his emotions and behavior and resulted in a substantial decrease in his endorsement of depressive symptoms (from 16 to 3 on the Pfizer, Prime MD Scale).

Service personnel are contacted either by telephone or in person at the time of follow-up and are assessed for PTSD, depression, alcohol usage, somatic complaints, days of poor physical and/or mental health, lost productivity, and satisfaction with health care. At the three-month PDHAT follow-up visit, SGT P endorsed a depressed mood but did not meet the full criteria for depression. He endorsed depressive symptoms at a level 12 (a score of 10 or above is of concern). PTSD symptoms were endorsed at a moderate level. Although he reported nine days of poor mental and physical health during the previous month, he only reported two days of lost productivity due to poor mental or physical health. He reported excellent satisfaction with his health care. At the six-month PDHAT follow-up visit, he endorsed depressive symptoms at a level 3 and did not meet the criteria for depression. He endorsed mild intrusive symptoms but did not meet criteria for PTSD. SGT P has returned to a light duty status while he continues to recover from his injuries.

## How Can Family and Friends Assist in the Healing Process

Getting a loved one to agree to accept help and finding support services for all family members are the first steps toward healing for the addicted person and the entire family.

When an addicted person is reluctant to seek help, sometimes family members, friends, and associates come together out of concern and love to confront the problem drinker. They strongly urge the person to enter treatment and list the serious consequences of not doing so, such as family breakup or job loss.

This is called "intervention." When carefully prepared and done with the guidance of a competent, trained specialist, the family, friends, and associates are usually able to convince their loved one—in a firm and loving manner—that the only choice is to accept help and begin the road to recovery.

People with alcohol- or drug-dependence problems can and do recover. Intervention is often the first step.

Children in families experiencing alcohol or drug abuse need attention, guidance, and support. They may be growing up in homes in which the problems are either denied or covered up.

These children need to have their experiences validated. They also need safe, reliable adults in whom to confide and who will support them, reassure them, and provide them with appropriate help for their age. They need to have fun and just be kids.

Families with alcohol and drug problems usually have high levels of stress and confusion. High-stress family environments are a risk factor for early and dangerous substance use, as well as mental and physical health problems.

It is important to talk honestly with children about what is happening in the family and to help them express their concerns and feelings. Children need to trust the adults in their lives and to believe that they will support them.

Children living with alcohol or drug abuse in the family can benefit from participating in educational support groups in their school student assistance programs. Those aged eleven and older can join Alateen groups, which meet in community settings and provide healthy connections with others coping with similar issues. Being associated with the activities of a faith community can also help.

If you're considering changing your drinking, you'll need to decide whether to cut down or to quit. It's a good idea to discuss different options with a doctor, a friend, or someone else you trust. Quitting is strongly advised if you:

- try cutting down but cannot stay within the limits you set
- have had an alcohol use disorder or now have symptoms
- have a physical or mental condition that is caused or worsened by drinking
- are taking a medication that interacts with alcohol
- are or may become pregnant

If you do not have any of these conditions, talk with your doctor to determine whether you should cut down or quit based on factors such as:

- family history of alcohol problems
- your age
- whether you've had drinking-related injuries
- symptoms such as sleep disorders and sexual dysfunction

### *Quitting Techniques*

Several proven treatment approaches are available. One size doesn't fit all, however. It's a good idea to do some homework on the Internet or at the library to find social and professional support options that appeal to you, as you are more likely to stick with them (see also Resources on the inside back cover). Chances are excellent that you'll pull together an approach that works for you.

#### SOCIAL SUPPORT

One potential challenge when people stop drinking is rebuilding a life without alcohol. It may be important to educate family and friends, develop new interests and social groups, find rewarding ways to spend your time that don't involve alcohol, and ask for help from others. When asking for support from friends or significant others, be specific. This could include not offering you alcohol, not using alcohol around you, giving words of support and withholding criticism, not asking you to take on new demands right now, and going to a group like Al-Anon. Consider joining Alcoholics Anonymous or another mutual support group (see Resources). Recovering people who attend groups regularly do better than those who do not. Groups can vary widely, so shop around for one that's comfortable. You'll get more out of it if you become actively involved by having a sponsor and reaching out to other members for assistance.

### PROFESSIONAL SUPPORT

Advances in the treatment of alcoholism mean that patients now have more choices and health professionals have more tools to help.

*Medications to treat alcoholism*. Newer medications can make it easier to quit drinking by offsetting changes in the brain caused by alcoholism. These options (naltrexone, topiramate, and acamprosate) don't make you sick if you drink, as does an older medication (disulfiram). None of these medications are addictive, so it's fine to combine them with support groups or alcohol counseling. A major clinical trial recently showed that patients can now receive effective alcohol treatment from their primary-care doctors or mental health practitioners by combining the newer medications with a series of brief office visits for support. See Resources for more information.

*Alcohol counseling*. "Talk therapy" also works well. There are several counseling approaches that are about equally effective—12-step, CBT, motivational enhancement, or a combination. Getting help in itself appears to be more important than the particular approach used, as long as it offers empathy, avoids heavy confrontation, strengthens motivation, and provides concrete ways to change drinking behavior.

*Specialized, intensive treatment programs*. Some people need more intensive programs. If you need a referral to a program, ask your doctor.

## Resources Available

There is help available on base and in your local community. Look in the Yellow Pages under Alcoholism for treatment programs and self-help groups. Call your county health department and ask for licensed treatment programs in your community. Keep trying until you find the right help for your loved one, yourself, and your family. Ask a family therapist for a referral to a trained interventionist or call the Intervention Resource Center at 1-888-421-4321.

Listed below are some useful websites if you are looking for more information about alcohol and drug use or about how to get help.

### *Substance Abuse*

#### VA PROGRAMS AND SERVICES

Abuse of substances such as alcohol, drugs, or tobacco can lead to increased risk of injuries, accidents, or physical and mental health problems. Although quitting is difficult, you do not have to do it alone.

- VA Substance Use Disorder (SUD) Program Locator: The program locator will help you find local VA SUD treatment programs.
- Effective treatments for substance use problems are available at VA. Available treatments address all types of problems related to substance use, from unhealthy use to life-threatening addictions. The "Summary of VA Treatment Programs for Substance Use Problems" page provides you with information on the treatment programs the VA uses.
- Smoking and tobacco use cessation: The VA's Office of Public Health and Environmental Hazards site provides information on quitting, preventing, and treating smoking and tobacco use for veterans, their families, and health professionals.
- MakeTheConnection.net: visit this site to view hundreds of stories from veterans of all service eras who have addressed their substance use and overcome mental health challenges. MakeTheConnection.net is a one-stop resource where veterans and their families and friends can privately explore information on mental health issues, hear fellow veterans and their families share their stories of resilience, and easily find and access the support and resources they need.
- Watch video testimonials from veterans who have found effective solutions to dealing with alcohol and drug problems, and to learn more about their experiences finding treatment and recovery.

#### OTHER RESOURCES

Al-Anon Family Groups: www.al-anon.org
Alateen: www.alateen.org
Adult Children of Alcoholics: www.adultchildren.org
Alcohol and Drug Abuse Information and Resources: www.alcoholanddrugabuse.com/

National Institute on Alcohol Abuse and Alcoholism: Frequently Asked Questions: http://www/niaaa.nij.gov
Substance Abuse Treatment Facility Locator: findtreatment.samhsa.gov/
Alcoholics Anonymous Homepage: www.alcoholics-anonymous.org/

### *Drugs*

Each year, drug and alcohol abuse contributes to the death of more than 120,000 Americans. According to the Office of National Drug Control Policy, drugs and alcohol cost taxpayers more than $328 billion annually in preventable health care costs, extra law enforcement, auto crashes, crime, and lost productivity.

Drug abuse is the use of drugs to get "high." It is a voluntary act, unlike drug addiction, which is involuntary. The addict is not able to stop using drugs unless there is intervention. Like alcoholism, drug addiction is a disease for which there is no cure.

Becoming addicted to drugs can occur extremely easily and very quickly, leaving the addict suffering from the severe effects of the drugs, and strong withdrawal effects if they do not take the drug. In order to cease the addiction a lot of support, help, and willpower is needed from both the addict and those around them.

The physical signs of a drug addiction can be quite varied depending on the drug used, the amount taken and the environment in which it is taken in. The early signs of a drug addiction can include mixed moods, sleepiness or excessive or unusual tiredness during the day, agitation, and paranoia. As the dependency develops the signs can change to being frequently distracted, depression, mixed mental states including psychosis, and a decrease in the ability to coordinate or perform tasks that are normally easy to complete. The degree of effect is variable between users and also on the substance of choice. Other very obvious signs are needle marks on the arms (though these can appear on other areas of the body once the veins in the arms have deteriorated and cannot be used any longer), but this only occurs in those who have been injecting the drugs. People who are normally nonsmokers are likely to suffer from breathlessness or coughing if they have been smoking drugs for long periods.

Although they are cheaper than they were a few decades ago, drugs are still an expensive commodity and most users struggle to keep up financially with their demand for their habit.

As the drug addiction develops the person is likely to become isolated from his or her usual family and friends and may get quite agitated when approached about this.

WHAT HAPPENS TO YOUR BRAIN WHEN YOU TAKE DRUGS?

Drugs are chemicals that tap into the brain's communication system and disrupt the way nerve cells normally send, receive, and process information. There are at least two ways that drugs are able to do this: (1) by imitating the brain's natural chemical messengers, and/or (2) by over stimulating the "reward circuit" of the brain. Some drugs, such as marijuana and heroin, have a similar structure to chemical messengers, called neurotransmitters, which are naturally produced by the brain. Because of this similarity, these drugs are able to "fool" the brain's receptors and activate nerve cells to send abnormal messages.

Other drugs, such as cocaine or methamphetamine, can cause the nerve cells to release abnormally large amounts of natural neurotransmitters, or prevent the normal recycling of these brain chemicals, which is needed to shut off the signal between neurons. This disruption produces a greatly amplified message that ultimately disrupts normal communication patterns.

Nearly all drugs, directly or indirectly, target the brain's reward system by flooding the circuit with dopamine. Dopamine is a neurotransmitter present in regions of the brain that control movement, emotion, motivation, and feelings of pleasure. The overstimulation of this system, which normally responds to natural behaviors that are linked to survival (eating, spending time with loved ones, etc.), produces euphoric effects in response to the drugs. This reaction sets in motion a pattern that "teaches" people to repeat the behavior of abusing drugs.

As a person continues to abuse drugs, the brain adapts to the overwhelming surges in dopamine by producing less dopamine or by reducing the number of dopamine receptors in the reward circuit. As a result, dopamine's impact on the reward circuit is lessened, reducing the abuser's ability to enjoy the drugs and the things that previously brought pleasure. This decrease compels those addicted to drugs to keep abusing drugs in order to attempt to bring their dopamine function back to normal. And, they may now require larger amounts of the drug than they first did to achieve the dopamine high—an effect known as tolerance.

Long-term abuse causes changes in other brain chemical systems and circuits as well. Glutamate is a neurotransmitter that influences the reward circuit and the ability to learn. When the optimal concentration of glutamate is altered by drug abuse, the brain attempts to compensate, which can impair cognitive function. Drugs of abuse facilitate nonconscious (conditioned) learning, which leads the user to experience uncontrollable cravings when they see a place or person they associate with the drug experience, even when the drug itself is not available. Brain-imaging studies of drug-addicted individuals show changes in areas of the brain that are critical to judgment, decision making, learning and memory, and behavior control. Together, these changes can drive an abuser to seek out and take drugs compulsively despite adverse consequences—in other words, to become addicted to drugs.

### WHY DO SOME PEOPLE BECOME ADDICTED, WHILE OTHERS DO NOT?

No single factor can predict whether or not a person will become addicted to drugs. Risk for addiction is influenced by a person's biology, social environment, and age or stage of development. The more risk factors an individual has, the greater the chance that taking drugs can lead to addiction. For example:

*Biology.* The genes that people are born with—in combination with environmental influences—account for about half of their addiction vulnerability. Additionally, gender, ethnicity, and the presence of other mental disorders may influence risk for drug abuse and addiction.

*Environment.* A person's environment includes many different influences—from family and friends to socioeconomic status and quality of life in general. Factors such as peer pressure, physical and sexual abuse, stress, and parental involvement can greatly influence the course of drug abuse and addiction in a person's life.

*Development.* Genetic and environmental factors interact with critical developmental stages in a person's life to affect addiction vulnerability, and adolescents experience a double challenge. Although taking drugs at any age can lead to addiction, the earlier that drug use begins, the more likely it is to progress to more serious abuse. And because adolescents' brains are still developing in the areas that govern decision making, judgment, and self-control, they are especially prone to risk-taking behaviors, including trying drugs of abuse.

### TREATMENTS

Before deciding on a program of drug treatment and support, the individual must be able to admit to having an addiction and actually want to overcome it. Positive thinking, willpower, and determination are fundamental to the success of following a drug-treatment plan.

Consideration should be given to whether a support group, individual counseling, or a combination of both will be beneficial. These types of therapy are useful as the therapists know what addiction is about, help you to determine the cause, and have a vast amount of advice regarding craving control, managing withdrawal, and how to restructure life without the addiction.

Find out about help lines and when they can be accessed, who runs them and what can be offered using them. Keep the list in close proximity at all times during the initial period of withdrawal and use these help lines when cravings are becoming too strong or anxieties are building up.

Allow for the "cold turkey" period. Warn family and close friends of what is happening and explain that it may cause distress to all those concerned. Exercise helps to ease symptoms of withdrawal so plan an exercise regime.

Overcoming an addiction is a very individual experience and a wide variety of resources may be needed to help break the drug addiction.

# 10

# Sleep Disturbance

## What Is It?

Many people who have been deployed for combat or peacekeeping experience sleep problems, for various reasons. Some individuals may suffer from nightmares related to the deployment, and wake up feeling terrified. Others may feel the need to stay awake to protect themselves from danger. For example, some service members who have been in combat feel a need to "stand guard" at night, rather than sleep. Individuals may also have poor sleep habits that lead to insomnia, such as extended napping or an irregular sleep schedule.

## The Extent of the Problem

Sleep disorder, or somnipathy, is a medical disorder and different to insomnia, which is difficulty falling and staying asleep. Serious sleep disorder, which can be caused by many things, can also lead to physical, mental, and emotional dysfunction.

Millions of people suffer from sleep disorders and more are diagnosed every year. Returning warriors are particularly prone to sleep disorders because of the additional stresses and tensions faced in a combat zone.

Common sleep disorders include:

- Primary insomnia: chronic difficulty in falling asleep and/or maintaining sleep when no other cause is found for these symptoms.
- Bruxism: involuntarily grinding or clenching of the teeth while sleeping.
- Delayed sleep phase syndrome (DSPS): inability to awaken and fall asleep at socially acceptable times but no problem with sleep maintenance, a disorder of circadian rhythms. (Other such disorders are advanced sleep phase syndrome (ASPS), non-twenty-four-hour sleep-wake syndrome (Non-24), and irregular sleep wake rhythm,

all much less common than DSPS, as well as the transient jet lag and shift work sleep disorder.)

- Hypopnea syndrome: abnormally shallow breathing or slow respiratory rate while sleeping.
- Narcolepsy: excessive daytime sleepiness (EDS) often culminating in falling asleep spontaneously but unwillingly at inappropriate times.
- Cataplexy: a sudden weakness in the motor muscles that can result in collapse to the floor.
- Night terror: *Pavor nocturnus*, sleep terror disorder: abrupt awakening from sleep with behavior consistent with terror.
- Parasomnias: disruptive sleep-related events involving inappropriate actions during sleep; sleep walking and night-terrors are examples.
- Periodic limb movement disorder (PLMD): sudden involuntary movement of arms and/or legs during sleep, for example kicking the legs; also known as nocturnal myoclonus. See also hypnic jerk, which is not a disorder.
- Rapid eye movement behavior disorder (RBD): acting out violent or dramatic dreams while in REM sleep (REM sleep disorder or RSD).
- Restless legs syndrome (RLS): an irresistible urge to move legs; RLS sufferers often also have PLMD.
- Situational circadian rhythm sleep disorders: shift work sleep disorder (SWSD) and jet lag.
- Sleep apnea, and mostly obstructive sleep apnea: obstruction of the airway during sleep, causing lack of sufficient deep sleep; often accompanied by snoring. Other forms of sleep apnea are less common. The air is blocked from entering into the lungs, causing the individual to unconsciously gasp for air. The individual will pause for an average of ten seconds in order to breathe. This is commonly found in overweight, middle-aged men but is also found in people who have suffered from stroke.
- Sleep paralysis: characterized by temporary paralysis of the body shortly before or after sleep; may be accompanied by visual, auditory, or tactile hallucinations. Not a disorder unless severe. Often seen as part of narcolepsy.
- Sleepwalking or *somnambulism*: engaging in activities that are normally associated with wakefulness (such as eating or dressing), which may include walking, without the conscious knowledge of the subject.
- Nocturia: A frequent need to get up and go to the bathroom to urinate at night. It differs from enuresis, or bed-wetting, in which the person does not arouse from sleep, but the bladder nevertheless empties.

## A Dread of Sleep

*How Does It Manifest Itself?*

Sleep disturbance can involve getting to sleep, waking up frequently during the night, and waking up too early. What are the treatment options? There are effective treatments for sleep problems. Choosing one that is right for you depends on the situation. Medications are available for quick, short-term relief of insomnia and nightmares. Some medications can be addictive, however, so check with your doctor to find out which is best for you.

Treatments for sleep disorders generally can be grouped into four categories:

- Behavioral and psychotherapeutic treatment
- Rehabilitation and management
- Medication
- Other somatic treatment

None of these general approaches is sufficient for all patients with sleep disorders. Rather, the choice of a specific treatment depends on the patient's diagnosis, medical and psychiatric history, and preferences, as well as the expertise of the treating clinician. Often, behavioral / psychotherapeutic and pharmacological approaches are not incompatible and can effectively be combined to maximize therapeutic benefits. Management of sleep disturbances that are secondary to mental, medical, or substance-abuse disorders should focus on the underlying conditions.

Medications and somatic treatments may provide the most rapid symptomatic relief from some sleep disturbances. Some disorders, such as narcolepsy, are best treated pharmacologically. Others, such as chronic and primary insomnia, may be more amenable to behavioral interventions, with more durable results.

Effective treatment begins with careful diagnosis using sleep diaries and perhaps sleep studies. Modifications in sleep hygiene may resolve the problem, but medical treatment is often warranted.

Special equipment may be required for treatment of several disorders such as obstructive apnea, the circadian rhythm disorders, and bruxism. In these cases, when severe, an acceptance of living with the disorder, however well managed, is often necessary.

Some "talk therapies" will help bring about long-term relief of sleep problems. Cognitive behavioral therapy targets your beliefs and behaviors that can make sleep problems worse. Sleep hygiene therapy helps people develop habits that can improve sleep. Breathing and relaxation therapies also may be used to help reduce muscle tension and promote sleep.

We are creatures of habit. Our sleep habits can either make sleeping easier or more difficult. The following ten suggestions have been shown to help reduce sleep problems:

1. *Keep bed only for sleep*—Do not watch TV, talk on the phone, review work, study, or solve problems while in bed. Go to bed only when you are drowsy and ready for sleep.
2. *If you don't fall asleep within thirty minutes, get up*—Go to another room and do something relaxing until you feel drowsy.
3. *"Wind down" before bedtime*—Do something calming, like light reading, listening to soothing music, praying, taking a warm bath, doing a crossword puzzle, or playing an enjoyable computer game before bedtime.
4. *Have a regular bedtime and rising time*—Go to sleep and wake up at the same time every day.
5. *Limit naps*—A mid-day nap as short as ten minutes can improve mood and mental performance. However, limit your nap to fifteen minutes and don't take it later than 4 pm, or the nap may interfere with your sleep cycle.
6. *Increase regular exercise*—Just not too close to bedtime.
7. *Decrease stimulants*—Avoid smoking, or drinking coffee or soda with caffeine in the afternoon or evening.
8. *Decrease alcohol*—Because alcohol causes mid-night awakenings, have no more than one serving of alcohol with dinner. Of course if you are in recovery from alcohol abuse, it is important to avoid alcohol entirely.
9. *Inspect your bedroom environment*—Is your bedroom dark and free of noise? Is your bed comfortable? Is the temperature comfortable? Do you feel safe and serene in your bedroom? If not, you can add images that are calming—a picture of your children, pet, an outdoor scene, a poem, or a prayer—to your room.
10. *Get help*—There are treatments that can help your sleep problems. If you continue to have sleep problems, see a trained sleep specialist to help identify what is the best treatment for you.

## What If I Am Having Nightmares?

After a traumatic event, many people experience nightmares. For some, nightmares may continue to repeat for a long period of time. During nightmares, you may feel like you are "reliving" the event, with the same fear, helplessness, or rage experienced during the original trauma. Nightmares are not a sign that you are "going crazy." They are a way of working through a trauma.

Some people try to avoid nightmares, by using drugs or alcohol, or by avoiding sleep altogether.

These "solutions" only lead to new problems, such as substance dependence and sleep deprivation. When you wake up from a nightmare, leave the bedroom and go to another room to get your bearings. It may take a while to reorient yourself to the present. Do something relaxing. If possible, reach out to someone who supports you. If you live with others, discuss the fact that you are having nightmares. Discuss ways in which you might want to handle the situation and share this chapter with them. A small percentage of sufferers act out their nightmare in their sleep. You may want to rearrange your bedroom so that you are safe. If you share your bed with a partner, you may need to make sure he or she is not in harm's way.

## How Can Family and Friends Assist?

Keep a sleep diary and record the individual's sleep patterns; this will be of great assistance if a visit to a sleep doctor is ordered. It should include what time the person went to bed and woke up, the total hours slept, and the number of times he or she woke during the night. It is also a good idea to record what food and drink was consumed before bed because this can have an effect on sleep quality. If you are sleeping with the person with the sleep disorder, record how loudly the person snores, whether breathing stops and how often, and how the person feels when he or she wakes.

As a family you can be supportive by trying to maintain a regular schedule—going to sleep and getting up at the same time every day, including the weekends. Most people don't get enough sleep in any case so make sure everyone can get at least seven to eight hours of sleep a night. Make sure the bedroom is dark, cool, and quiet. If necessary, use heavy curtains or shades to block out light. Have the person wear an eye mask if it helps and even ear plugs, and turn off smart phones and any computers in the room as the light they emit can interfere with the body's internal clock and disturb sleep.

## Resources Available

National Center for Posttraumatic Stress Disorder: www.ptsd.va.gov
National Alliance for the Mentally Ill: http://www.nami.org/Learn-More/Mental-Health-Conditions/Related-Conditions/Sleep-Disorders
Stanford University Center for Excellence in the Diagnosis and Treatment of Sleep Disorders: http://sleep.stanford.edu

# 11

# Sexual Trauma and Hazing

## What Is It?

"Military sexual trauma" (MST) is the term that the US Department of Veterans Affairs (VA) uses to refer to sexual assault or repeated, threatening sexual harassment that occurred while the veteran was in the military. It includes any sexual activity where someone is involved against his or her will—he or she may have been pressured into sexual activities (for example, with threats of negative consequences for refusing to be sexually cooperative or with implied faster promotions or better treatment in exchange for sex), may have been unable to consent to sexual activities (for example, when intoxicated), or may have been physically forced into sexual activities. Other experiences that fall into the category of MST include unwanted sexual touching or grabbing; threatening, offensive remarks about a person's body or sexual activities; and/or threatening or unwelcome sexual advances.

Both women and men can experience MST during their service. All veterans seen at Veterans Health Administration (VHA) facilities are asked about experiences of sexual trauma because it is known that any type of trauma can affect a person's physical and mental health, even many years later. It is also known that people can recover from trauma. VA has free services to help veterans do this. You do not need to have a VA disability rating (be "service connected") to receive these services and may be able to receive services even if you are not eligible for other VA care. You do not need to have reported the incident(s) when they happened or have other documentation that they occurred.

## The Extent of the Problem

Information about how commonly MST occurs comes from VA's universal screening program. Under this program, all veterans seen at VHA facilities are asked whether they experienced sexual trauma during their military service; veterans who respond "yes" are asked if they are interested in learning about MST-related services available. Not every veteran who responds "yes" needs or is necessarily interested in treatment. It's important to note that rates obtained from VA screening cannot be used to make any estimate of the rate of MST among all those serving in the US military, as they are drawn only from veterans who have chosen to seek VA health care. Also, a positive response does not indicate that the perpetrator was a member of the military.

About one in five women and one in a hundred men seen in VHA respond "yes" when screened for MST. Though rates of MST are higher among women, because of the disproportionate ratio of men to women in the military there are actually only slightly fewer men seen in VA that have experienced MST than there are women.

## How Does It Manifest Itself?

When overwhelmed by strong emotions, the body and mind sometimes react by shutting down and becoming numb. As a result, veterans may have difficulty experiencing loving feelings or feeling some emotions, especially when upset by traumatic memories. Like many of the other reactions to trauma, this emotional numbing reaction is not something the veteran is doing on purpose.

### *How Can MST Affect Veterans?*

It's important to remember that MST is an experience, not a diagnosis or a mental health condition in and of itself. Given the range of distressing sexually related experiences that veterans report, it is not surprising that there are a wide range of emotional reactions that veterans have in response to these events. Even after severely distressing experiences, there is no one way that everyone will respond—the type, severity, and duration of a veteran's difficulties all vary based on factors like whether the veteran has a prior history of abuse, the types of responses from others the veteran received at the time of the experiences, and whether the experience happened once or was repeated over time. For some veterans, experiences of MST may continue to affect their mental and physical health, even many years later.

Some of the difficulties both female and male survivors of MST may have include:

*Strong emotions:* feeling depressed; having intense, sudden emotional reactions to things; feeling angry or irritable all the time

*Feelings of numbness:* feeling emotionally "flat," difficulty experiencing emotions like love or happiness

*Trouble sleeping:* trouble falling or staying asleep; disturbing nightmares

*Difficulties with attention, concentration, and memory:* trouble staying focused; frequently finding their mind wandering; having a hard time remembering things

*Problems with alcohol or other drugs*: drinking to excess or using drugs daily; getting intoxicated or "high" to cope with memories or emotional reactions; drinking to fall asleep

*Difficulty with things that remind them of their experiences of sexual trauma:* feeling on edge or "jumpy" all the time; difficulty feeling safe; going out of their way to avoid reminders of their experiences; difficulty trusting others

*Difficulties in relationships:* feeling isolated or disconnected from others; abusive relationships; trouble with employers or authority figures

*Physical health problems:* sexual difficulties; chronic pain; weight or eating problems; gastrointestinal problems

Among users of VA health care, medical record data indicates that diagnoses of posttraumatic stress disorder (PTSD) and other anxiety disorders, depression and other mood disorders, and substance-use disorders are most frequently associated with MST.

Fortunately, people can recover from experiences of trauma, and VA has services to help veterans do this.

Services available to veterans include:

- All veterans seen in VA health care are asked whether they experienced MST and all treatment for physical and mental health conditions related to experiences of MST is free for both men and women.
- Every VA health care facility has a designated MST coordinator who serves as a contact person for MST-related issues. This person can help veterans find and access VA services and programs. He or she may also be aware of state and federal benefits and community resources that may be helpful.
- Every VA health care facility has providers knowledgeable about treatment for the aftereffects of MST. Many have specialized outpatient mental health services focusing on sexual trauma. Vet Centers also have specially trained sexual-trauma counselors.
- Nationwide, there are programs that offer specialized sexual-trauma treatment in residential or inpatient settings. These are programs for veterans who need more intense treatment and support.

- To accommodate veterans who do not feel comfortable in mixed-gender treatment settings, some facilities have separate programs for men and women. All residential and inpatient MST programs have separate sleeping areas for men and women.

To receive free, confidential treatment for mental and physical health conditions related to MST, *veterans do not need to be service connected* (have a VA disability rating). Veterans may be able to receive this benefit even if they are not eligible for other VA care. Veterans do not need to have reported the incident(s) when they happened or have other documentation that they occurred.

*Intimacy Issues*

At first, many service members feel disconnected or detached from their partner and/or family. You may be unable to tell your family about what happened. You may not want to scare them by speaking about the war. Or maybe you think that no one will understand. You also may find it's hard to express positive feelings. This can make loved ones feel like they did something wrong or are not wanted anymore. Sexual closeness may also be awkward for a while. Remember, it takes time to feel close again.

Intimacy is a combination of emotional *and* physical togetherness. It is not easily reestablished after stressful separations creating an emotional disconnect.

Partners may also experience high or low sexual interest causing disappointment, friction or a sense of rejection. In due time, this may pass, but present concerns may include hoping one is still loved, dealing with rumors or concern about faithfulness, concern about medications that can affect desire and performance, and expected fatigue and alterations in sleep cycles.

*What are the treatment options?*

It is essential to get proper counseling whether you are the victim of sexual abuse or experiencing emotional issues that are affecting your sex life.

While MST can be a very difficult experience, recovery is possible. Treatment can help improve your quality of life by focusing on strategies for managing emotions and memories or, for veterans who are ready, involve actually talking about their MST experiences in depth.

## How Can Family and Friends Assist?

Many veterans who are the victims of sexual trauma do not tell family and friends. It is important to understand why revealing something like this can be so difficult. Victims in the military cannot leave their jobs and they have to continue working alongside their attacker often in very dangerous circumstances. Until recently there were no real channels for making confidential complaints about MST so many victims remained silent lest they affect their chances of promotion. Equally important, even when a formal complaint was made, the perpetrator more often than not simply received a slap on the wrist.

That is why many victims remain silent and need the love and understanding that families and friends can provide.

## Resources Available

At VA, veterans can receive free, confidential treatment for mental and physical health conditions related to MST. You may be able to receive this MST-related care even if you are not eligible for other VA services. To receive these services, you do not need a VA service-connected disability rating, to have reported the incident when it happened, or have other documentation that it occurred.

Knowing that MST survivors may have special needs and concerns, every VA health care facility has an MST coordinator who can answer any questions you might have about VA's MST services. VA also has a range of other services available to meet veterans where they are at in their recovery:

*Other Resources*

MakeTheConnection.net. Visit this site to view stories of veterans who have overcome MST. MakeTheConnection.net is a one-stop resource where veterans and their families and friends can privately explore information on mental health issues, hear fellow veterans and their families share their stories of resilience, and easily find and access the support and resources they need.

After Deployment. The website afterdeployment.org provides a program designed to give support to service members who are healing after having experienced sexual trauma.

MyDuty.mil. If you are an active duty service member and have been a victim of military sexual assault (or know someone who has), MyDuty.mil provides information and guidance on your reporting options and rights.

DoD Safe Helpline. The DoD Safe Helpline is a crisis support service for members of the US Department of Defense (DoD) community affected by sexual assault. Through the Safe Helpline, you can "click, call or text" to receive anonymous one-on-one advice, support, and information

24/7. You can go to www.safehelpline.org for a live chat or to view resources. From anywhere in the world, you can call 877-995-5247 or text your zip code or base/installation name to 55-247 inside the United States (202-470-5546 outside the United States) to get the contact information for your nearest sexual assault response coordinator.

## Hazing

Hazing is another subject that every branch of the military takes very seriously and is working diligently to stamp out. Hazing is often regarded as a required rite of passage but it can lead to serious assault, both physical and sexual, and in some cases even death.

There were a number of high-profile hazing cases in 2011. Two members of the military committed suicide after allegedly being hazed in separate attacks. One was a Marine and the other a soldier, both serving in Afghanistan.

While all branches of the military condemn hazing and have policies against it, the practice continues. Now Congress has started a series of hearings to examine the scope of the problem and what the Pentagon is doing to stop it.

Marine Corps Commandant General Jim Amos has called for a full review of the Corp's fifteen-year-old policy on hazing, ordered that all hazing allegations be tracked and investigated, and has told senior officers to be more aggressive in tackling claims of abuse. "Regardless of the form it takes, hazing is always unacceptable. It destroys our Marines' confidence and trust in their fellow Marines and in unit leadership, thus undermining unit cohesion and combat readiness," Amos wrote in a letter to the Corps.

Unfortunately, there are few details about how widespread the problem is. When DoD officials were asked by members of Congress for hazing statistics, they were unable to produce any figures. The Pentagon is trying to get this information from each branch of the military although it is not clear whether every service documents hazing allegations.

In evidence to the House committee on March 22, 2012, US Coast Guard Master Chief Petty Officer Michael Leavitt said:

> As the Master Chief Petty Officer of the Coast Guard ensuring our personnel are treated with dignity and respect is a responsibility I take very seriously.
>
> The Coast Guard does not tolerate hazing. Hazing is contrary to our core values of honor, respect and devotion to duty and the nature of our missions.
>
> The Coast Guard has published a clear and unambiguous policy prohibiting hazing, including requirements for initial training of all military service members, as well as annual training thereafter. When hazing has occurred our policy requires that offenders are held accountable. All Commanding

> Officers are required to investigate any hazing incident and initiate appropriate action to hold those accountable for hazing misconduct, as well as to ensure accountability within the chain of command if hazing was condoned.

The Coast Guard defines hazing as any physical, verbal, or psychological conduct in which a military member causes another military member to suffer or to be exposed to any cruel, abusive, humiliating, oppressive, demeaning, or harmful activity, regardless of the perpetrator's and recipient's service or rank. Soliciting or coercing another to conduct such activity also constitutes hazing.

The Coast Guard's hazing policy is found in the Discipline and Conduct Manual. The policy defines hazing, outlines roles and responsibilities, mandates annual training, and lists consequences. Furthermore, the policy clearly states that consent by the hazing victim does not obviate accountability of either the persons doing the hazing or the Command that condones or facilitates a hazing incident. Hazing incidents can be adjudicated under the provisions of the Uniform Code of Military Justice. Depending on the severity of the hazing incident, and how it is disposed of, punishment may include confinement, fines, reduction in rank, and/or punitive discharge from the Coast Guard.

Similar to hazing, prohibited harassment policy is found in the Coast Guard's Civil Rights Manual. Prohibited harassment is defined as including, but not limited to, unwelcome conduct, whether verbal, nonverbal, or physical conduct that has the purpose or effect of unreasonably interfering with an individual's work performance or creating an intimidating, offensive, or hostile environment on the basis of an individual's protected status, which includes: race, color, religion, sex, national origin, age, disability, genetic information, sexual orientation, marital status, parental status, political affiliation, or any other basis protected by law. While hazing and prohibited harassment are similar, each type of case is reported and acted upon in a different manner. In each case, perpetrators are subject to prompt disciplinary action, including discharge and other actions authorized under the Uniform Code of Military Justice. Incidents of prohibited harassment are processed in accordance with the Coast Guard's Antiharassment and Hate Incident Procedures and as a complaint of employment discrimination pursuant to the Coast Guard's Civil Rights Manual.

"Hazing typically occurs in connection with unofficial, unsupervised initiations or other informal 'rites of passage' that are not authorized in the Coast Guard. Traditional ceremonies are permitted but must be conducted with proper command sanction and oversight to prevent harassment of any kind," said Leavitt. "Assault and Sexual Assault are specific illegal acts defined in the Uniform Code of Military Justice and could potentially be committed during incidences of hazing. Incidences of assault or sexual assault occurring as part of hazing are aggravating factors, and therefore carry the potential for more severe consequences to offenders."

In February 2010, the Coast Guard Investigative Service concluded a nearly year-long investigation into allegations that former crew members onboard Coast Guard Cutter VENTUROUS home ported in St. Petersburg, Florida, had engaged in hazing between the summer of 2007 and the spring of 2009.

As a result of the investigation, seven Coast Guardsmen were tried by courts-martial for the most serious misconduct related to hazing activities onboard the Coast Guard Cutter VENTUROUS between 2007 and 2009. Several other crew members received administrative action under the Uniform Code of Military Justice for less serious infractions. According to court records, the hazing took place in the berthing areas of the ship while underway and was done unbeknownst to senior leadership. The seven courts-martial resulted in five members receiving confinement or restrictions of up to five months, six members being reduced in pay grade, three members forfeiting pay, one member being discharged, and one member receiving a Bad Conduct Discharge.

In addition to the hazing on VENTUROUS, there have been three additional courts-martial stemming from hazing incidents since 2009. These included cases at Station Cape Disappointment, SECTOR Mobile, and SECTOR San Francisco. Two of the cases are in final legal review. The third case is set for trial in April of this year.

Twenty-three Coast Guardsmen have been identified as the "targets," or victims of serious hazing misconduct. Eighteen, or 78 percent, of the victims are Caucasian. Other victims are distributed across many racial profiles to include one Asian American, one African American, one Hispanic, one Hawaiian Islander, and one Native American/Alaska Native. "Juniority" of rank appears to be the common characteristic of the victims of serious hazing misconduct.

### *Hazing Victim Racial Profiles*

No data is available to determine if hazing was or was not a contributing factor in any suicide that has occurred in the Coast Guard. Throughout the past ten years, the number of suicides has remained fairly consistent, averaging six active duty and reservist suicides per year, which represents roughly 0.01 percent of our workforce.

Sergeant Major of the Army Raymond Chandler said, "My overall message to the force is the Army profession. I talk about what it means to be a professional, how Soldiers should conduct themselves, and more importantly, how they should treat each other."

Master Chief Petty Officer of the Navy Rick West told the committee that "people are absolutely our most precious asset. Their individual

**Table 11.1 The Results of One Survey Showing the Breakdown by Race of Victims of Serious Hazing Misconduct in the Coast Guard**

| *White* | *Asian* | *Black* | *Hispanic* | *Other* | *Total* |
|---|---|---|---|---|---|
| 78% (18) | 4% (1) | 4% (1) | 4% (1) | 4% (1) | 23 |

success and the Navy's collective mission accomplishment lie in our ability to provide an environment that promotes inclusiveness and a validated sense of value to the team," he said.

"Hazing unequivocally destroys these ideas and is not tolerated in your Navy," West said. "It is inconsistent to our core values of honor, courage and commitment, and detrimental to individual esteem and unit cohesion."

Sergeant Major of the Marine Corps Michael P. Barrett stated, "Hazing is not a part of our service culture or who we are. . . . Hazing fosters a climate of maltreatment and cruelty—concepts inconsistent with our core values. As an institution, the only way that the Marine Corps can exist, survive and thrive is through fostering a climate where Marines have every opportunity for participation and advancement in accordance with their talents, backgrounds, culture and skills."

### *How to Tackle the Problem*

Preventing hazing can best be achieved by addressing two key elements: training and leadership.

Awareness and support of the hazing policies are emphasized by senior leadership through the use of communications to all ranks and other formal and informal outreach efforts. For example, the Coast Guard Commandant as well as the Pacific and Atlantic Area Commanders released official messages regarding the responsibility of all Coast Guardsmen to comply with the Coast Guard's zero tolerance hazing policy. The Commandant included a requirement in his message that all commanding officers and officers in charge read the message at the next quarters or appropriate muster to ensure his expectations and intent are clear.

Training courses held at the Leadership Development Center for Prospective Commanding Officers and Boat Forces Command Cadre include segments on hazing, aim to ensure future leaders understand and enforce the policy.

Hazing prevention cannot be achieved purely by the actions of military leaders. All personnel must understand that hazing will not be tolerated and no one may consent to being hazed. To ensure awareness throughout the military workforce, most branches provide initial training on hazing to all new recruits and require annual unit training.

# 12

# SUICIDE

Suicide is when someone purposely takes his or her own life. Many people think about committing suicide at some time in their lives, especially in times of extreme stress or depression, but most don't follow through. Suicide, like depression, affects people of all ages and backgrounds.

War experiences and war-zone stress reactions, especially those caused by personal loss, can lead a depressed person to think about hurting or killing him- or herself. If you or someone you know is feeling this way, take it seriously, and get help.

Usually, people who commit suicide think their situation is totally hopeless. In this state of mind, death can seem like the only option. But, there are always other options and there is hope. The quickest way to get help is to call one of the national suicide-prevention lifelines available 24/7 at: **1-800-273-TALK** (1-800-273-8255) or **1-800-SUICIDE** (1-800-784-2433).

## The Extent of the Problem

According to the Department of Defense (DoD) Suicide Prevention and Risk Reduction Committee's (SPARRC) Preventing Suicide Network, every year, thirty thousand Americans take their own lives. While the suicide rate for military members is substantially lower than their civilian counterparts, it is still a significant cause of death for many of our military.

However, since the start of the Iraq War in 2003, the rate of suicide among US soldiers has soared, according to a study from the US Army Public Health Command.

The study, an analysis of data from the Army Behavioral Health Integrated Data Environment, shows an 80 percent increase in suicides among Army personnel between 2004 and 2008. The rise parallels increasing rates of depression, anxiety, and other mental health conditions in soldiers, the study said.

The high number of suicides are "unprecedented in over 30 years of U.S. Army records," according to the authors of the study, which was published in the journal *Injury Prevention*. Based on the data and the timing of the increase in suicide rates, the authors calculated that about 40 percent of the Army's suicides in 2008 could be associated with the US military escalation in Iraq.

"This study does not show that U.S. military operations in Iraq and Afghanistan cause suicide. . . . This study does suggest that an Army engaged in prolonged combat operations is a population under stress, and that mental health conditions and suicide can be expected to increase under these circumstances," said Dr. Michelle Chervak, one of the study's authors, a senior epidemiologist at the US Army Public Health Command.

In 2007 and 2008 alone, 255 active duty soldiers committed suicide. The vast majority of the suicides since 2004 were by men; and 69 percent had seen active combat duty. Nearly half were between ages eighteen and twenty-four. And 54 percent of those who committed suicide were from among the lower ranks of enlisted personnel. The study found that suicide rates were higher among soldiers who had been diagnosed with a mental illness in the year before their death.

Soldiers who had been diagnosed with major depression were more than eleven times as likely to commit suicide, and suicide was ten times more likely among those with anxiety. More than 25 percent of the soldiers who took their lives had been diagnosed with adjustment disorder, a term for the immediate emotional fallout from proximity to stressful events.

## How Does It Manifest Itself?

These findings play into the known general risk factors for suicide including:

- Stressful life events when combined with depression or other risk factors. However, many people have stressful life events and are not at risk for suicide.
- A family history of mental disorder or substance abuse, especially if it includes violence—physical or sexual
- A prior suicide attempt
- A family history of suicide
- Exposure to the suicidal behavior of others, such as family members, peers, or media figures
- Depression, mental disorders, and substance abuse (more than 90 percent of the people who commit suicide have these risk factors)

- Having firearms in the home
- Incarceration

Most suicide attempts are not harmless bids for attention, but are expressions of extreme distress. A person who appears suicidal should not be left alone and needs immediate mental health treatment.

Most mental health problems were first identified during visits with primary-care doctors, not with mental health professionals. Tell your doctor if you notice any of the following:

- Talking about wanting to hurt or kill yourself
- Trying to get pills, guns, or other things that you could use to harm yourself
- Talking or writing about death, dying, or suicide
- Hopelessness
- Rage, uncontrolled anger, seeking revenge
- Saying or feeling there's no reason for living
- Acting in a reckless or risky way
- Feeling trapped, like there's no way out

### How Can Family and Friends Assist

Suicide hotlines are free and confidential, are staffed by trained counselors, and have information about support services that can be of assistance. Suicide hotlines should be contacted when:

The sadness is overwhelming, or there are thoughts of hopelessness or suicide.

There is concern about someone who may be experiencing these feelings.

There is interest in suicide prevention, treatment, and service referrals.

### What to Do If Someone Says He or She Is Thinking about Suicide

When someone is at risk for suicide, take immediate action by doing the following:

Tell someone immediately! Never promise to keep thoughts about suicide a secret.

Take the person's concerns seriously, and listen without judging.

Tell the person what will be done to help, such as not discussing the issue with coworkers unless it's on a need-to-know basis. A need-to-know basis might include command or someone else who can help.

Limit the person's access to firearms or other lethal means of committing suicide (this may require getting additional assistance).

It may be necessary to involve others to help, such as military law enforcement, 911, or others that can help such as friends or family members.

Help the person get to a health care professional. Give him or her the number to a mental health professional, chaplain, or a counselor in your installation, or to the national suicide prevention hotlines at **1-800-273-TALK** (1-800-273-8255) or **1-800-SUICIDE**, or (1-800-784-2433). Military OneSource (1-800-342-9647; www.militaryonesource.com) is another resource. Stay with the person until he or she has contacted help.

If the person refuses to get help, don't keep suicide thoughts a secret. Tell a friend, family member, professional, or supportive leader who can find the person help.

## Resources Available

### *Military Programs*

#### DOD SPARRC PREVENTING SUICIDE NETWORK

The DoD SPARRC Preventing Suicide Network is a resource center aimed at providing authoritative and problem-specific information about suicide prevention. SPARRC aims to help military personnel, family, and friends who are concerned about someone who may be at risk for suicide, so that they can locate tailored resources about suicide prevention. The program also educates the public, mental health clinicians and other professionals about suicide-prevention education and research, and it promotes active collaboration among professionals and consumers in all segments of suicide prevention treatment, policy, education, and research. The SPARRC website (www.suicideoutreach.org) provides information on what to look for and what to do to help someone who you think may be dealing with thoughts of suicide. Up-to-date information is available so that you can become more educated about suicide and to see what researchers are currently doing. The site also provides service-specific resources which are listed below:

- Air Force

  Air Force Suicide Prevention Program: www.af.mil/SuicidePrevention.aspx

- Army

US Army Center for Health Promotion and Preventive Medicine Suicide Prevention Program: http://phc.amedd.army.mil/topics/healthyliving/bh/Pages/SuicidePreventionEducation.aspx

- Coast Guard

  Coast Guard Suicide Awareness Program: www.uscg.mil/worklife/suicide_prevention.asp

- Marine Corps

  Marine Corps Community Services Suicide Prevention Program: www.usmarines.com/us-marines-suicide-prevention

- Navy

  Navy Suicide Prevention Program: http://www.public.navy.mil/bupersnpc/support/21st_Century_Sailor/suicide_prevention/Pages/default.aspx

### *Government Suicide Prevention Programs*

#### NATIONAL SUICIDE PREVENTION LIFELINE

The National Suicide Prevention Lifeline is a national, twenty-four-hour, toll-free suicide-prevention service available to anyone in suicidal crisis who is seeking help. You can get help by dialing 1-800-273-TALK (8255), and then pressing 1 to be routed to the Veterans Hotline. This will then transfer you to the closest possible provider of mental health and suicide-prevention services. To learn more about the Lifeline, local crisis centers, and other resources, go to: http://www.healthypeople.gov/2020/prevention-portal-508/initiative/national-strategy-for-suicide-prevention.

#### NATIONAL STRATEGY FOR SUICIDE PREVENTION (NSSP)

The NSSP provides facts about suicide, recent publications, and resources designed to spread knowledge of the seriousness of suicides. A resource from the site can display state-specific suicide prevention programs. For more information, visit: mentalhealth.samhsa.gov/suicideprevention.

#### NATIONAL INSTITUTE OF MENTAL HEALTH (NIMH)

This portion of the NIMH website contains information on statistics and prevention of suicide in the United States, resources that cover suicide and related mental illnesses, in addition to connections to ongoing clinical trials involved in suicide. To see this and more information, go to: www.nimh.nih.gov/health/topics/suicide-prevention/index.shtml.

CENTER FOR DISEASE CONTROL AND PREVENTION (CDC)

Suicide facts, risk factors, warning signs, and prevention strategies are described to provide you with a better understanding of how to recognize if you or someone you care for may be dealing with thoughts of suicide. To learn more, visit: www.cdc.gov/ncipc/dvp/Suicide/default.htm.

### *Support Organizations for the Prevention of Suicide*

AMERICAN FOUNDATION FOR SUICIDE PREVENTION

The site offers assistance to people whose lives have been affected by suicide and offers support and opportunities to become involved in prevention. Learn more at: www.afsp.org.

MEDLINEPLUS

MedlinePlus provides information about warning signs and how to deal with them, as well as how to cope with suicide. Go to: www.nlm.nih.gov/medlineplus/suicide.html.

NATIONAL ASSOCIATION FOR PEOPLE OF COLOR AGAINST SUICIDE (NOPCAS)

NOPCAS gives information on depression and other brain disorders, coping methods for survivors, and suicide-prevention and intervention tips. Visit the website at: www.nopcas.org/resources.

MENTAL HEALTH AMERICA DEPRESSION SCREENING

The Mental Health America website describes symptoms and treatments for depression and provides a free, confidential depression-screening test. (Note: This screening test is not intended to provide a diagnosis for clinical depression, but may help identify any depressive symptoms and determine whether a further evaluation by a medical or mental health professional is necessary): http://depressionscreen.org.

SUICIDE AWARENESS VOICES OF EDUCATION (SAVE)

SAVE offers depression and suicide information, strategies for coping with loss, and resource links. Learn more at: www.save.org.

### MENTAL HEALTH SELF-ASSESSMENT PROGRAM (MHSAP)

The MHSAP program is designed for you to identify your own symptoms and access assistance for PTSD, depression, generalized anxiety disorder, alcohol use, and bipolar disorder before a problem becomes serious. For more information, go to: www.mentalhealthscreening.org/military/index.aspx.

### CENTRE FOR SUICIDE PREVENTION

The website for the Centre for Suicide Prevention describes what to do if you or someone you care for is suicidal, provides resources for suicide prevention, and answers frequently asked questions about suicide. Visit the website at: www.suicideinfo.ca/csp/go.aspx?tabid=1.

### SUICIDE PREVENTION ADVOCACY NETWORK

The Suicide Prevention Advocacy Network offers support to suicide survivors (those who have lost a loved one to suicide and those who have attempted suicide) and leverages to advance public policies that help prevent suicides. Visit the website at: www.spanusa.org.

# 13

# FAMILIES

The reunion of a family after a separation can be just as stressful as the separation itself. If your family has experienced some strain or tension during a reunion, you are not alone. You may have wondered why an occasion that is "supposed" to be so romantic and exciting should turn out less than perfect.

From the moment you are separated from the person you care about, you may begin to build up an image of that person in your mind. You may fantasize about how wonderful everything will be when you are together again.

You may remember the members of your family as they appear in the photograph in your wallet—the picture perfect all-American family. A similar process is happening with the spouse and children. The missing member may be placed on a pedestal as the warrior out defending the country. Memories of everyday life such as making ends meet, occasional disagreements, and disciplining the children, begin to fade from everyone's mind. The reunion is seen as the solution to all problems. "Once we are together again, everything will be perfect." However, reality rarely has a chance to live up to the high expectations you have set in your minds.

This is not meant to be a forecast of "doom and gloom." Homecomings can be very happy occasions as long as all family members make an effort to be as realistic as possible. If the tendency to not pick up after oneself around the house occurred before the separation, that habit probably has not miraculously disappeared. If a weight problem existed prior to the separation, do not expect a fifty-pound loss to have occurred during the separation. If one of the children was experiencing problems at school, do not expect the problem to disappear at reunion time.

Talking to one another and working through the everyday challenges that family life presents is what is important. This does not all have to be accomplished on the day of the family reunion. Give yourselves some time to enjoy one another. Everyone needs to get reacquainted before problem-solving begins.

## Dangers and Threats

The primary source of support for the returning soldier is likely to be his or her family. We know from veterans of the Vietnam War that there can be a risk of disengagement from family at the time of return from a war zone. We also know that emerging problems with acute stress disorder and posttraumatic stress disorder can wreak havoc with the competency and comfort the returning soldier experiences as a partner and parent. While the returning soldier clearly needs the clinician's attention and concern, that help can be extended to include his or her family as well. Support for the veteran and family can increase the potential for the veteran's smooth immediate or eventual reintegration back into family life and reduce the likelihood of future, more damaging problems.

## The Extent of the Problem

If one or both partners are identifying high tension or levels of disagreement, or the clinician is observing that their goals are markedly incompatible, then issues related to safety need to be assessed and plans might need to be made that support safety for all family members. Couples who have experienced domestic violence and/or infidelity are at particularly high risk and in need of more immediate support. When couples can be offered a safe forum for discussing, negotiating, and possibly resolving conflicts, that kind of clinical support can potentially help to reduce the intensity of the feelings that can become dangerous for a family. Even support for issues to be addressed by separating couples can be critically valuable, especially if children are involved and the parents anticipate future coparenting.

## How Does It Manifest Itself?

Stress reactions in a returning war veteran may interfere with the ability to trust and be emotionally close to others. As a result, families may feel emotionally cut off from the service member. The veteran may feel irritable and have difficulty with communication, making him or her hard to get along with. He or she may experience a loss of interest in family social activities. The veteran may lose interest in sex and feel distant from his or her spouse.

Traumatized war veterans often feel that something terrible may happen "out of the blue" and can become preoccupied with trying to keep themselves and family members safe.

Just as war veterans are often afraid to address what happened to them, family members also may avoid talking about the trauma or related problems.

They may avoid talking because they want to spare the veteran further pain, or because they are afraid of his or her reaction. Family members may feel hurt, alienated, or discouraged because the veteran has not overcome the effects of the trauma and may become angry or feel distant from the veteran.

## What Are the Options?

If the veteran is living at home, the clinician can meet with the family and assess with them their strengths and challenges and identify any potential risks. Family and clinician can work together to identify goals and develop a treatment plan to support the family's reorganization and return to stability in coordination with the veteran's work on his or her own personal treatment goals.

Inpatient hospitalization could lengthen the time returning personnel are away from their families, or it could be an additional absence from the family for the veteran who has recently returned home. It is important to the ongoing support of the reuniting family that clinicians remain aware that their patient is a partner and/or parent. Family therapy sessions, in person or by phone if geographical distance is too great, can offer the family a forum for working toward meeting their goals. The potential for involving the patient's family in treatment will depend on their geographic proximity to the treatment facility. Distance can be a barrier, but the family can still be engaged through conference phone calls or visits.

## How Can Family and Friends Assist?

The primary source of support for the returning soldier is likely to be his or her family. Families can help the veteran avoid withdrawal from others. Families can provide companionship and a sense of belonging, which can help counter feelings of separateness and difference from other people. They can provide practical and emotional support for coping with life stressors.

If the veteran agrees, it is important for family members to participate in treatment. It is also important to talk about how the posttrauma stress is affecting the family and what the family can do about it. Adult family members should also let their loved ones know that they are willing to listen if the service member would like to talk about war experiences. Family members should talk with treatment providers about how they can help in the recovery effort.

### *Self-Care Suggestions for Families*

- Take time to listen to all family members and show them that you care.
- Spend time with other people. Coping is easier with support from caring others, including extended family, friends, church, or other community groups.
- Join or develop a support group.
- Take care of yourself. Family members frequently devote themselves totally to those they care for, and in the process, neglect their own needs. Watch your diet, exercise, and get plenty of rest. Take time to do things that feel good to you.
- Try to maintain family routines, such as dinner together, church, or sports outings.

## Homecoming after Deployment: Dealing with Changes and Expectations

A NATIONAL CENTER FOR PTSD FACT SHEET

*Ilona Pivar, PhD*

With deployment comes change. Knowing what to expect and how to deal with changes can make homecoming more enjoyable and less stressful. Below are some hints you might find helpful.

### *Expectations for Service Personnel*

- You may miss the excitement of the deployment for a while.
- Some things may have changed while you were gone.
- Face-to-face communication may be hard at first.
- Sexual closeness may also be awkward at first.
- Children have grown and may be different in many ways.
- Roles may have changed to manage basic household chores.
- Spouses may have become more independent and learned new coping skills.
- Spouses may have new friends and support systems.
- You may have changed in your outlook and priorities in life.

- You may want to talk about what you saw and did. Others may seem not to want to listen. Or you may not want to talk about it when others keep asking.

*Expectations for Spouses*

- Your partner
    - May have changed.
    - May be used to the open spaces of the field, may feel closed in.
    - May be overwhelmed by noise and confusion of home life.
    - May be on a different schedule of sleeping and eating (jet lag).
    - May wonder if he or she still fits into the family.
    - May want to take back all the responsibilities he or she had before deployment.
    - May feel hurt when young children are slow to hug them.

*What Children May Feel*

- Babies less than one year old may not know you and may cry when held.
- Toddlers (one to three years) may hide from you and be slow to come to you.
- Preschoolers (three to five years) may feel guilty over the separation and be scared.
- School age children (six to twelve years) may want a lot of your time and attention.
- Teenagers (thirteen to eighteen years) may be moody and may appear not to care.
- Any age children may feel guilty about not living up to your standards.
- Some may fear your return ("Wait until mommy/daddy gets home!").
- Some may feel torn by loyalties to the spouse who remained.

*Tips for Service Personnel*

- Support good things your family has done.
- Take time to talk with your spouse and children.
- Make individual time for each child and your spouse.
- Go slowly when reestablishing your place in the family.
- Be prepared to make some adjustments.
- Romantic conversation can lead to more enjoyable sex.
- Make your savings last longer.

- Take time to listen and to talk with loved ones.
- Go easy on partying.

*Tips for Spouses for Reunion*

- Avoid scheduling too many things.
- Go slowly in making adjustments.
- You and your soldier may need time for yourself.
- Remind soldier he or she is still needed in the family.
- Discuss splitting up family chores.
- Stick to your budget until you've had time to talk it through.
- Along with time for the family, make individual time to talk.
- Be patient with yourself and your partner.

*Tips for Reunion with Children*

- Go slowly. Adapt to the rules and routines already in place.
- Let the child set the pace for getting to know you again.
- Learn from how your spouse managed the children.
- Be available to your child, both with time and with your emotions.
- Delay making changes in rules and routines for a few weeks.
- Expect that the family will not be the same as before you left; everyone has changed.
- Focus on successes with your children; limit your criticisms.
- Encourage children to tell you about what happened during the separation.
- Make individual time for each child and your spouse.

*Caregiver Support*

Your military spouse, son, or daughter may have an injury or illness, and, as a result, may require a considerable amount of care once released from the hospital. Many family members of recovering service members have found themselves in this role. Sometimes this role is temporary while the service member recovers. Other times, as is sometimes the case with traumatic brain injuries, you may be in the role of caregiver for a much longer time.

As a new caregiver, you may be concerned about your abilities to handle the task, wondering if you can cope with the change in your role, fearful of what is ahead, and you may be mourning the loss of the way things were before the injury or illness. You may feel overwhelmed and not know where to turn for help.

There are a variety of resources that can help you. You are not alone. As a caregiver, you may be relied upon to help your loved one with a broad range of activities, including cooking, eating, bathing, and dressing. You may need to take care of paying his or her bills and making medical decisions. A variety of services are available to help you assist a disabled service member or veteran.

### ASSESSING YOUR NEEDS

In order to know what assistance you need, you may find it helpful to ask yourself the following questions:

What type of help does my husband / wife / son / daughter need in order to live as independently as possible? (Consider the following options: companionship, housekeeping, grocery shopping, and transportation to the military treatment facility.)
When do you need help?
What help can be provided?
How much money is available to pay for outside resources? Do you have additional insurance to help offset the cost of these services?
Are any friends or family willing to pitch in? What help have they offered?

### CAREGIVING CAN TAKE A TOLL ON YOU

Research suggests that the physical and emotional demands on caregivers put them at greater risk for health problems:

Caregivers are more at risk for infectious diseases, such as colds and flu, and chronic diseases, such as heart problems, diabetes, and cancer.

Depression is twice as common among caregivers compared to noncaregivers.

### CAREGIVERS AND DEPRESSION

If you find yourself feeling sad, alone, overwhelmed, or angry, you may be experiencing depression. It's not unusual for caregivers to experience mild to more severe depression.

While the caregivers do everything they can to give the best possible care to their injured loved one, they often place their own physical and emotional needs second, third—even last. After a while, this can cause anger, sadness, isolation, and exhaustion. Once these feeling are identified, guilt often results.

Thoughts like, "How can I blame him? It's not his fault that he was injured," or "She's my 'baby' and needs me. How can I put my needs ahead of hers?" can cause monumental guilt, driving you to work through the negative feelings and, once again, put your needs after the injured person's needs.

Everyone has negative feelings, but if they don't go away, or if they leave you drained of energy and you find yourself angry at your loved one, or crying all the time, they may be signs that you are depressed. Ignoring the feelings will not make them go away.

### SYMPTOMS OF DEPRESSION

The symptoms of depression are different for everyone and only a mental health care professional is qualified to tell you if you are clinically depressed.

There are symptoms that may indicate depression. Some are listed below:

- Difficulty staying focused
- Significant weight loss or gain from a change in eating habits
- Sleeping much more or having difficulty sleeping
- Constant fatigue
- Lack of interest in the activities and people you once enjoyed
- Feelings of hopelessness
- Thoughts of hurting yourself
- Thoughts of killing yourself
- Constant disorders (headache, stomachache, etc.) that do not respond to treatment

It's essential to get help for your depression. Without assistance, your quality of life will continue to decline.

### HOW YOU CAN COMBAT DEPRESSION

First, you should consult with a trained health or mental health professional. If you think that you are depressed, a good place to get help is to start with your family doctor. If you feel uncomfortable saying that you think you are depressed, tell your health professional that you "feel blue" or "feel down." They will know what to ask. Be prepared to answer questions like:

- Why do you think you feel this way?
- When did the symptoms start?
- How long have you felt this way?
- How often do you use alcohol or drugs to feel better?
- Do you have family members who suffer from depression?
- Do you have a friend or someone with whom you can confide?

Besides the health professional's treatment, there are ways you can help yourself. In no way are these suggestions meant to be replacements for professional care. But taking care of yourself in the following ways may help ease some of your depression.

- Set realistic goals. Examples might include going to bed thirty minutes earlier; loading the dishwasher in the morning; making a simple, quick dinner rather than a more elaborate meal.
- Try to be with other people—confide in a friend.
- Do something enjoyable—work in thirty minutes of exercise, go to a movie, meet a friend for coffee.
- Break larger tasks into smaller ones and accomplish what you can.
- Try to think positive thoughts.
- Let your friends and family help you.
- Eat balanced meals.

Help is always as close as your friends, family, and the network of those in a similar situation. Remember, there are others who are in a similar situation as you. Reach out to them through support groups, in person, or online. You may find that sharing experiences will help you in a number of ways.

*Community Care Options*

Community care programs and services, along with eligibility requirements, vary in different states, counties, and communities. Many of these agencies and organizations are located on the National Resource Directory website.

Informal support offered by friends, family, religious communities, local organizations, neighbors, and others can share the responsibilities of caregiving, including doing household chores, providing emotional support for you and your loved one, and helping the recovering service member maintain a healthy level of social and recreational activity.

In this case, making a list of your helpers and their phone numbers will be an invaluable source of support for routine help or in times of emergency. Information and referral helps you by identifying your local resources.

## Resources Available

*American Red Cross*. While providing services to 1.4 million active duty personnel and their families, the Red Cross also reaches out to more than 1.2 million members of the National Guard and the Reserves and their families who reside in nearly every community in America. Red Cross workers in hundreds of chapters and on military installations brief departing service members and their families regarding available support services and explain how the Red Cross may assist them during the deployment. See www.redcross.org.

Both active duty and community-based military can count on the Red Cross to provide emergency communications that link them with their families back home, access to financial assistance, counseling and assistance to veterans. Red Cross Service to the Armed Forces personnel work in 756 chapters in the United States, on fifty-eight military installations around the world, and with our troops in Kuwait, Afghanistan, and Iraq.

*Military OneSource* is a "one stop shop" for information on all aspects of military life. From information about financial concerns, parenting, relocation, emotional well-being, work, and health, to many other topics, Military OneSource can provide a wealth of information. There are many informative topics on the website specific to wounded service members and families. See: www.militaryonesource.com.

*Army Morale Welfare and Recreation.* Army recreation programs. See: www.armymwr.com.

*Army OneSource.* Website of choice for Army families providing accurate, updated articles and information on various topics. See: www.myarmyonesource.com

*Azalea Charities.* Provides comfort and relief items for soldiers, sailors, airmen and Marines sick, injured, or wounded from service in Iraq and Afghanistan. It purchases specific items requested by military medical centers, VA medical centers and Fisher House rehabilitation facilities each week. It also provides financial support to CrisisLink, a hotline for wounded soldiers and their families, and Hope for the Warriors, special projects for wounded soldiers. See: www.azaleacharities.com.

*Blue Star Mothers of America* is a nonprofit organization of mothers who now have, or have had, children honorably serving in the military. Their mission is "supporting each other and our children while promoting patriotism." See: www.bluestarmothers.org.

*The Military Family Network.* One nation, one community, making the world a home for military families. See: www.emilitary.org.

*Military Connection.* Comprehensive military directory providing information on job postings, job fairs, and listings. See: www.militaryconnection.com.

*Military Homefront.* Website for reliable quality of life information designed to help troops, families, and service providers. See: www.militaryhomefront.dod.mil.

*National Military Family Association.* NMFA's primary goals are to educate military families concerning their rights, and benefits and services available to them; to inform them regarding the issues that affect their lives; and to promote and protect the interests of military families by influencing the development and implementation of legislation and policies affecting them. Great publications online such as "Resources for Wounded and Injured Service Members and Their Families" and "Your Service Member Your Army—A Parent's Guide" are available. See: www.militaryfamily.org.

*The National Remember Our Troops Campaign* works to recognize military service members and their families by providing an official US Blue or Gold Star Service Banner. The Star Service Banner displayed in the window of a home is a tradition dating back to World War I. See www.nrotc.org.

*Strategic Outreach to Families of All Reservists* helps Reservist families reduce their stress and prepare for the possibility that their Reservist or Guard member may exhibit symptoms of trauma from serving in a combat zone. The goal of SOFAR is to provide a flexible and diverse range of psychological services that fosters stabilization and aids in formulating prevention plans to avoid crises, and helps families to manage acute problems effectively when they occur. See: www.sofarusa.org.

# 14

# Homelessness and Mental Health

An estimated one-third of the adult homeless population have donned a uniform and served in the military. The US Department of Veterans Affairs (VA) estimates that roughly sixty-seven thousand veterans are homeless on any given night, with perhaps twice that experiencing homelessness at some period over the course of a year. Many other veterans are considered near homeless or at risk of becoming homeless.

VA states the nation's homeless veterans are predominantly male, with roughly 5 percent being female. The majority of them are single; come from urban areas; and suffer from mental illness, alcohol and/or substance abuse, or cooccurring disorders.

America's homeless veterans have served in World War II, the Korean War, Cold War, Vietnam War, Grenada, Panama, Lebanon, Afghanistan and Iraq (OEF/OIF), and the military's antidrug cultivation efforts in South America. Nearly half of homeless veterans served during the Vietnam era. Two-thirds served our country for at least three years, and one-third were stationed in a war zone.

Roughly 56 percent of all homeless veterans are African American or Hispanic, despite only accounting for 12.8 percent and 15.4 percent of the US population, respectively.

About 1.5 million other veterans, meanwhile, are considered at risk of homelessness due to poverty, lack of support networks, and dismal living conditions in overcrowded or substandard housing. Nearly half a million (467,877) veterans were severely rent burdened and paying more than 50 percent of their income for rent. More than half (55 percent) of veterans with severe housing-cost burden fell below the poverty level and 43 percent were receiving food stamps.

In addition to the complex set of factors influencing all homelessness—extreme shortage of affordable housing, livable income, and access to health care—a large number of displaced and at-risk veterans live with lingering effects of posttraumatic stress disorder (PTSD) and substance abuse, which are compounded by a lack of family and social-support networks.

A top priority for homeless veterans is secure, safe, clean housing that offers a supportive environment free of drugs and alcohol.

Although "most homeless people are single, unaffiliated men . . . most housing money in existing federal homelessness programs, in contrast, is devoted to helping homeless families or homeless women with dependent children," as is stated in the study "Is Homelessness a Housing Problem?" (Wright and Rubin 1997, 947).

VA is taking decisive action to end veteran homelessness in five years, it announced in December, 2011. All veterans at risk for homelessness or attempting to exit homelessness must have easy access to programs and services including prevention, housing support, treatment, employment, and job training.

VA also announced it will make $100 million in grants available to community agencies across the country to prevent nearly forty-two thousand veterans and their families from falling into homelessness or to quickly return them to stable housing. The funds are offered for fiscal year 2012 through VA's Supportive Services for Veteran Families (SSVF) program, a homeless-prevention and rapid rehousing program.

"The problems that lead to homelessness begin long before Veterans and their families are on the streets," said Secretary of Veterans Affairs Eric K. Shinseki (2010). "By putting more resources into prevention services for those at risk of becoming homeless, we will continue to help more Veterans and their families turn their lives around."

Last year, VA provided $60 million through the SSVF program to community providers, which will affect nearly twenty-two thousand people through eighty-five nonprofit community agencies in forty states and the District of Columbia. The program provides community organizations with funding for counseling, training, education assistance, direct time-limited financial assistance, transportation, child care, rent, utilities, and other services aimed at preventing homelessness or providing homes for participating veterans and family members.

Being homeless does not mean the veteran has a mental health problem, although many of them do. However, being homeless does mean that many veterans do not get adequate medical attention and proper counseling so that any conditions they might have often go untreated.

Dr. Keith Harris, who is the VA National Director of Clinical Operations, Mental Health Homeless and Residential Rehabilitation Treatment Programs, recognizes the social disconnect in homeless veterans:

> One of the most serious symptoms of homeless people is the lack of a sense of control. We use a phrase to capture our approach to treatment: "I create what happens to me." We find that this approach helps homeless people move away from a past-focused sense of victimhood to a more active, future-oriented role in molding the conditions of their lives.
>
> The percentages of homeless Veterans with substance use or psychiatric issues is telling. In the most recent annual report of the Health Care for Homeless Veterans program, which is VA's outreach and case management program, it reported that 64% had a diagnosis of drug *or* alcohol dependence."
>
> Another 57% had a diagnosis of serious mental illness. Serious mental illness is defined as having a psychiatric diagnosis that falls into one of the following categories: schizophrenia, other psychotic disorder, mood disorders and PTSD.
>
> It's also significant that 82% had a diagnosis of *either* drug *or* alcohol dependence *or* serious mental illness. (U.S. Department of Veterans Affairs, 2010)

(These statistics vary depending on the program reports, as the programs target different issues and acuity levels.)

Given the large majority of homeless veterans with substance-use or psychiatric issues, VA has placed a large emphasis on treating these issues within its homeless programs. Veterans are treated within the homeless programs, and / or referred to specialty care as needed. The majority of veterans report significant improvement in these areas upon leaving VA homeless programs.

"When you consider the causes of homelessness, in addition to lack of employment or income, often times you find mental health issues and substance use issues or a combination of both. So in working to help people find housing and jobs, programs to support mental health and substance use treatment work hand in hand" (U.S. Department of Veterans Affairs, 2010).

## Programs

The US Department of Housing and Urban Development (HUD) and VA continue to work together to end veterans' homelessness. Through tools like HUD-VASH, HUD and VA are making some real progress towards this goal. HUD and VA have housed about twenty times as many veterans in the last two years than ever before—twenty-five thousand more veterans since the beginning of the program.

The Recovery Act's Homelessness Prevention and Rapid Rehousing Program (HPRP) has been another important resource toward the progress made so far. Together with the HEARTH Act, HUD and VA will continue providing HPRP's rapid rehousing and preventive services to veterans who are returning from Iraq and Afghanistan. This means that for the first time veterans will have a true continuum of assistance—from prevention and outreach, to emergency shelter, transitional housing and rapid rehousing, to permanent supportive housing.

## Community Homelessness Assessment, Local Education, and Networking Groups for Veterans (CHALENG)

At the local level, VA medical centers designate CHALENG point-of-contacts (POC) who are responsible for coordinating local CHALENG efforts. These CHALENG POCs work with local agencies throughout the year to coordinate services for homeless veterans. Ninety-two percent of POC sites that had a nearby HUD Continuum of Care planning group participated in the local Continuum of Care planning efforts.

- Nationwide, VA homeless programs have over five thousand interagency collaborative agreements (formal and informal) to serve homeless veterans.
- 3,118 outreach sites (such as shelters, soup kitchens, welfare offices, or other locations where homeless persons may be found) were accessed.
- About one-fifth (21 percent) of sites indicated they have an on-campus housing program operated by a community partner.
- 95 percent of sites that prioritized permanent housing in their action plan reported success, due mainly to the nationwide expansion of the HUD-VASH program.
- CHALENG POC action addresses priority needs such as permanent, emergency, and transitional housing; job finding; dental care; transportation; VA disability/pension; job training; food; and drop-in center or day program.
- Although the overall consumer ranking may indicate that a particular need is a high-ranking unmet need, this result can vary widely by the current homelessness status of the veteran. For example, child care ranks as the highest unmet need overall, however veterans in shelters or on the streets do not rank child care as a "top ten" unmet need.
- VA's highly integrated health care model has made medical and mental health treatment readily accessible to veterans. Veterans rank these services as highly met needs. However, not all health care needs are ranked as being met. Veteran consumers who are literally homeless (defined in this report as sleeping in the streets, shelters, or areas unfit for human habitation) or those in permanent

housing, rank dental care as the third and first highest unmet needs, respectively.
- Overall, family and legal concerns rank as the fourth-highest ranked unmet needs, ahead of permanent, transitional, and emergency housing.

## Resources Available

VA offers a range of programs and services designed to help homeless veterans live as self-sufficiently and independently as possible, including outreach, clinical assessment and referral to medical treatment, employment assistance, and supported permanent housing.

Visit the VA Homeless Veterans website (www1.va.gov/homeless) to find more information on:

- Prevention services (including the National Call Center for Homeless Veterans, Veteran Justice Outreach, and Supportive Services for Low Income Veterans)
- Housing support services (including HUD's and VA's Supported Housing Program [HUD-VASH] and The Grant and Per Diem Program)
- Treatment (including Healthcare for Homeless Veterans Program (HCHV), Healthcare for Reentry (HCRV), and Drop-in Centers and Domiciliary Care Program)
- Employment/job training (compensated work therapy)
- Benefits/other services
- Other resources

You can also find a homeless veteran coordinator/program by state.

- MakeTheConnection.net: visit this site to view hundreds of stories from veterans of all service eras who have overcome mental health challenges. MakeTheConnection.net is a one-stop resource where veterans and their families and friends can privately explore information on mental health issues, hear fellow veterans and their families share their stories of resilience, and easily find and access the support and resources they need.
- Watch video testimonials from veterans who have overcome mental health challenges, and to find information on homelessness and resources for support.

*Caregivers*

Family Caregiver Alliance—National Center on Caregiving: www.caregiving.org/

National Alliance for Caregiving: www.caregiver.org

Health and Human Services—Medicare Site—Caregiving Exchange: www.medicare.gov/campaigns/caregiver/caregiver.html

# 15

# Resilience

## What Is It?

Resilience is the ability to cope and recover from stress and life-changing events. It helps us adjust to a normal life after deployment and it provides the strength to overcome adversities and illness, especially when there is an accompanying strong and loving support group.

With homecoming, you may need to relearn how to feel safe, comfortable, and trusting with your family. Developing resilience will help you do this and make you a stronger person in the process.

You must get to know one another again. Good communication with your partner, children, parents, siblings, friends, coworkers, and others is the key. Give each other the chance to understand what you have been through. When talking as a family, be careful to listen to one another. Families work best when there is respect for one another and a willingness to be open and consider alternatives.

## Self-Help? Tips for Feeling Better

It's fine for you to spend some time alone. But if you spend too much time alone or avoid social gatherings, you will be isolated from family and friends. You need the support of these people for a healthy adjustment. You can help yourself to feel better by:

- Getting back to regular patterns of sleep and exercise.
- Pursuing hobbies and creative activities.
- Planning sufficient R&R and intimate time.
- Trying relaxation techniques (meditation, breathing exercises) to reduce stress.
- Learning problems to watch out for and how to cope with them.
- Striking a balance between staying connected with former war buddies and spending individual time with your partner, kids, other family members, and friends.

- Communicating more than the "need-to-know" bare facts.
- Talking about your war zone experiences at a time and pace that feels right to you
- Not drinking to excess, or when you're feeling depressed or to avoid disturbing memories. Drink responsibly, or don't drink.
- Creating realistic workloads for home, school, and work.

## Steps to Assuming Normal Routines

Soon after your return, plan to have an open and honest discussion with your family about responsibilities. You all need to decide how they should be split up now that you're home. It's usually best to take on a few tasks at first and then more as you grow accustomed to being home. Be willing to compromise so that both you and your family members feel that needs are understood and respected.

Try to reestablish a normal sleep routine as quickly as possible. Go to bed and get up at the same time every day. Do not drink to help yourself sleep.

You might try learning some relaxation techniques, such as deep breathing, yoga, or meditation.

### *Important Points to Remember*

- Readjusting to civilian life takes time—don't worry that you're experiencing some challenges. Find solutions to these problems. Don't avoid.
- Take your time adding responsibilities and activities back into your life.
- Reconnect with your social supports. This may be the last thing you feel like doing, but do it anyway. Social support is critical to successful reintegration.
- Review BATTLEMIND to understand where some of your automatic behaviors come from.
- Remind your loved ones that you love them.
- Realize that you need to talk about the experiences you had during deployment.
- If you can't talk to family or friends, be sure to talk to a chaplain or counselor.

### *Red Flags*

You now know the reactions that are normal following deployment to war. But sometimes the behaviors that kept you alive in the war zone get you on the wrong track at home. You may not be able to shut them down after you've returned home safely. Some problems may need outside assistance to solve.

Even serious post-deployment psychological problems can be treated successfully and cured. Being able to admit you have a problem can be tough:

- You might think you should cope on your own.
- You think others can't help you.
- You believe the problem(s) will go away on their own.
- You are embarrassed to talk to someone about it.

If your reactions are causing significant distress or interfering with how you function, you will need outside assistance. Things to watch for include:

- Relationship troubles—frequent and intense conflicts, poor communication, inability to meet responsibilities
- Work, school, or other community dysfunction—frequent absences, conflicts, inability to meet deadlines or concentrate, poor performance
- Thoughts of hurting someone, or yourself
- If you get assistance early, you can prevent more serious problems from developing. If you delay seeking help because of avoidance or stigma, your problems may actually cause you to lose your job, your relationships, and your happiness. Mental and emotional problems can be managed or treated, and early detection is essential.

## How Can Family and Friends Assist?

Getting help when you need it is crucial in building your resilience. Beyond caring family members and friends, people often find it helpful to turn to:

*Self-help and support groups.* Such community groups can aid people struggling with hardships such as the death of a loved one. By sharing information, ideas, and emotions, group participants can assist one another and find comfort in knowing that they are not alone in experiencing difficulty.

*Books and other publications.* Many people who have successfully managed adverse situations such as surviving cancer have written about their experiences. These stories can motivate readers to find a strategy that might work for them personally.

*Online resources.* Information on the web can be a helpful source of ideas, though the quality of information varies among sources.

## Safe Helpline, the Ground-Breaking Crisis Support Service for Members of the Military

The DoD has launched the *Safe Helpline*, a groundbreaking crisis-support service for members of the DoD community affected by sexual assault. Safe Helpline provides live, one-on-one support, and information to the worldwide DoD community.

The service is confidential, anonymous, secure, and available worldwide, 24/7 by click, call, or text—providing victims with the help they need, anytime, anywhere. Specially trained Safe Helpline staff provides help three ways.

*Online Helpline*

Safe Helpline provides live, confidential help through a secure instant-messaging format at SafeHelpline.org. The website also contains vital information about recovering from and reporting a sexual assault.

*Telephone Helpline*

Safe Helpline also provides live, confidential help over the phone—just call. The telephone helpline is available from anywhere, anytime—twenty-four hours a day, seven days a week, worldwide: 877-995-5247. The phone number is the same inside the United States or via the Defense Switched Network (DSN). When calling from DSN, there are four toll-free area codes (800, 888, 866, and 877) as DSN area codes to enable a direct dialing capability. DSN users can dial US toll-free numbers by simply dialing 94 + the ten-digit toll-free number.

The telephone helpline staff even transfer callers to installation and base Sexual Assault Response Coordinators (SARCs), Military OneSource, the National Suicide Prevention Lifeline, and civilian sexual-assault service providers. The phone number is the same in the United States and worldwide via the DSN.

*Text for Info*

Safe Helpline can provide you with referrals by text to your mobile phone. You can text your zip code, installation or base name to 55-247 (inside the United States) or 202-470-5546 (outside the United States), and Safe Helpline will text back contact information for the SARC on your installation or base. You can also search for help here.

Safe Helpline services (click, call, or text) are administered by the DoD Sexual Assault Prevention and Response Office (SAPRO) and are operated by RAINN (Rape, Abuse and Incest National Network), the nation's largest anti-sexual-violence organization. However, your information will remain confidential. RAINN will not share your name or any other personally identifying information with SAPRO or your chain of command.

RAINN created and operates the National Sexual Assault Hotline (800.656.HOPE) in partnership with over 1,100 local rape crisis centers nationwide. RAINN also runs the National Sexual Assault Online Hotline (online.rainn.org). Together, the hotlines have helped more than 1.6 million people since 1994.

For many people, using their own resources and the kinds of help listed above may be sufficient for building resilience. At times, however, an individual might get stuck or have difficulty making progress on the road to resilience.

*A licensed mental health professional.* A psychologist can assist people in developing an appropriate strategy for moving forward. It is important to get professional help if you feel like you are unable to function or perform basic activities of daily living as a result of a traumatic or other stressful life experience.

Different people tend to be comfortable with somewhat different styles of interaction. A person should feel at ease and have good rapport in working with a mental health professional or participating in a support group.

## Resources Available

American Psychological Association: www.apa.com
National Resilience Resource Center-University of Minnesota: http://www.nationalresilienceresource.com
The Institute for the Study of Human Resilience: www.bu.edu/cpr/

# 16

# HEALTH AND WELLNESS

## What Is It?

Wellness is a proactive approach to being healthy. It encompasses what you eat and drink, how you exercise and how you manage stress. It usually involves lifestyle changes but the bottom line is a healthier, longer, and happier (stress-free) life—and that has got to be something worth going for.

## Self-Help

Wellness research shows that Americans who take care of themselves and manage their lifestyles are healthier, more productive, have fewer absences from work, and make fewer demands for medical services. An article published in the *Journal of the American Medical Association* indicated that, in one study, the "wellness" approach resulted in a 17 percent decline in total medical visits and a 35 percent decline in medical visits for minor illness.

Eat sensibly, exercise properly, and manage stress and you will achieve physical, emotional, and psychological wellness.

### *Sensible Eating*

Maintaining a healthy weight means balancing the number of calories you eat with the calories your body uses or burns.

If you maintain your weight, you are "in balance." You are eating close to the same number of calories that your body is using. Your weight will remain stable.

If you are gaining weight, you are eating more calories than your body is using. These extra calories will be stored as fat, and you will gain weight.

If you are losing weight, you are eating fewer calories than you are using. Your body is using its fat storage cells for energy, so your weight is decreasing.

A simple way to know if you are at a healthy weight is to know your body mass index (BMI). Here is a link to a BMI table: www.move.va.gov/download/NewHandouts/Miscellaneous/M06_BMIChart.pdf.

## BMI GUIDELINES

Underweight = BMI less than 18.5
Normal weight = BMI of 18.5–24.9
Overweight = BMI of 25–29.9
Obesity = BMI of 30 or greater

Being a healthy, normal weight is good for you and will help you prevent and control many diseases and conditions. Being overweight or obese increases your risk for diabetes, high blood pressure, cholesterol problems, heart disease, gallbladder disease, female health disorders, arthritis, some types of cancer, and sleep apnea.

Eat wisely and choose a variety of low-calorie, high-nutrition foods and beverages in the basic food groups. Select foods that limit your intake of fats, cholesterol, added sugars, salt, and alcohol.

## EATING AT HOME

- Take charge. Plan for healthy meals and snacks.
- Never eat out of boxes, cartons, or bags unless they are single-serving packages.
- Put food on a plate or in a bowl. Then, you can see how much you are eating.
- Use smaller plates, bowls, or glasses.
- Be careful of tasting or nibbling while you cook.
- Sit at the table to eat.
- Fix your plate in the kitchen and bring it to the table to eat. Leave the serving bowls, pots, or containers in the kitchen so you won't be tempted to eat more.
- Let leftovers be leftovers.
- Eating while watching television, working on the computer, or talking on the phone may cause you to overeat.
- Take time to relax and enjoy your food! You can find pleasure from both preparing and eating.

## EATING WELL ON A BUDGET

Healthy eating does not have to be expensive. Here are some tips for keeping your calories and budget in balance:

- Plan your weekly menu in advance. Make a grocery list and stick to it.
- Checkout the weekly ads for the supermarkets with the best sales.
- Clip coupons. Choose only ones that you will use and are a real cost-saver.
- Try not to shop when you are hungry.
- Compare store and generic brands for the best buy.
- Take advantage of sales. Cook in bulk and freeze or use leftovers for future meals.
- Stretch costly meals (like meat dishes) by adding lots of vegetables.
- Read food labels to get the best nutrition and the most value for your money.
- Choose fresh fruit and vegetables that are in season. Visit your local farmers market for produce.
- Fruit and vegetables are canned or frozen at the peak of freshness. Choose fruit that is frozen, unsweetened, or canned in its own juice.
- Beans, peas, eggs, canned tuna (packed in water), and peanut butter are good sources of protein and good buys.
- Grow your own vegetables, fruit, or herbs.

## SNACK ATTACK

*50–75 Calories*

- One medium piece of fresh fruit or one-half to one cup of cut fruit
- One cup raw vegetables such as sliced peppers, mushrooms, and tomatoes with two tablespoons hummus or fat-free salad dressing
- Two saltine crackers with two teaspoons peanut butter

*100–125 Calories*

- One cup nonfat, sugar-free yogurt with one-half cup fresh or frozen, unsweetened berries
- One plain rice cake with one-half tablespoon peanut butter and one-half banana, sliced
- One-half cup cottage cheese with one-quarter cup berries
- One slice of toast with one-quarter cup 1 percent cottage cheese, sprinkled with cinnamon
- Fruit smoothie with three-fourths cup nonfat yogurt and one-half cup fruit
- One ounce of pretzels
- Three fig cookies

*150–200 Calories*

- One-half small whole wheat pita with one ounce of low-fat cheese and one-half cup cooked or fresh vegetables
- One small corn tortilla wrapped around one piece of low-fat string cheese with one tablespoon of salsa
- One slice bread with mustard, two slices turkey breast, and a slice of tomato
- One small–medium apple with one tablespoon peanut butter
- One-fourth cup nut and raisin mix
- One cereal bar or reduced-fat granola bar
- Four cups of low-fat, air-popped or microwave popcorn

## SPECIAL OCCASION EATING

Special occasions such as parties, celebrations, or holiday meals can pose risks for overeating. Here are some tips:

- Consider the weight loss you have achieved so far and what you have done to get to this point. Is splurging really worth it?
- Avoid drinking alcoholic beverages as they are empty calories and make it harder for you to avoid temptation.

*Be Prepared* Eat a small meal or snack before the special occasion so that you are less hungry.

Fill up ahead of time on water or other low-calorie beverages.

- Don't Deny Yourself

  Go ahead and have a taste of those special foods, but limit your portion sizes. Eat these special foods slowly and enjoy every morsel.

  Choose low calorie munchies such as crunchy vegetables for balance.

- Keep Your Hands and Mouth Occupied

  Focus on the conversation and having a good time rather than the eating. Get out on the dance floor!

  Chew gum or have a mint.

  Keep a glass in your hand containing a low-calorie drink. It is hard to overeat if your hands are busy.

*Don't Go*

- If the only way you can handle temptation is to avoid it, don't go.

*Restaurant Tips*

- Choose restaurants you know will have healthy options. Many restaurants have websites. Check out menus in advance.
- You don't have to eat it all—ask for part of your meal to be packaged to go.

*Food Preparation*

- Don't be afraid to ask how items are prepared.
- Ask for low-fat cooking spray or little or no butter or oil to be used.
- Look for choices that are roasted, poached, steamed, baked, and grilled rather than sautéed, deep fried, or pan fried. If it is sautéed, ask for wine or lemon juice to be used. If you do eat fried foods, remove any breading and skin.
- Ask for sauces on the side.

*Appetizers—Choose Soup or Salad*

- Choose clear broth soups or tomato-based soups.
- Avoid cream-based choices such as a bisque, chowder, or cheese soup.
- Avoid salads that contain fried foods. Ask for poultry, meat, or seafood to be grilled.
- Ask for fat-free or low-fat dressing. Always ask for the dressing to be put on the side, not tossed in the salad. Try vinegar or lemon juice on your salad.
- Leave off extras like croutons, cheese, egg, nuts, fried noodle strips, and so on.

*Entrée*

- When choosing vegetarian choices, avoid cheese, cream, and so on.
- Select skinless poultry, preferably white meat, and lean cuts of beef and pork such as tenderloin, London broil, or filet mignon. Avoid ribs, prime rib, and other marbled meats.

*Sides*

- Choose colorful vegetables.
- Skip the creamed vegetables or those that have cheese.
- Be adventurous. Try something new instead of the old stand-by of French fries.
- Choose fresh fruit or a tossed salad over potato salad, coleslaw, macaroni salad, and so on.

*Beverages*

- Drink plenty of water or low-calorie sugar-free beverages with your meal.
- Consider low-fat or skim milk.

*Dessert*

- Order fresh fruit.
- Choose a small bowl of low-fat ice cream, sorbet, sherbet, gelatin, or a piece of angel food cake.
- If you order dessert, split it with someone else.

*Bread*

- If bread is too tempting for you, ask your server not to bring the basket to your table.
- Limit bread to one to two slices per meal. Choose baked bread, rolls, and saltine crackers instead of croissants, biscuits, and cornbread.
- Leave off butter or margarine. For toast, ask for it "dry."
- Eat slowly. Take plenty of time to savor the food's flavor. Enjoy yourself!

*Water—Drink Up!* Water has major functions in the body. Drinking enough water is an important part of a healthy lifestyle and a successful weight management program. Here are some tips:

- Sometimes, we feel hungry when we are actually dehydrated.
- Don't wait for thirst! Sip throughout the day.
- Always keep a water bottle with you.
- Take "water breaks" throughout the day.
- Drink decaffeinated beverages or plain water with meals.
- Don't skip the water fountain—always take a sip.

How much water do we need?

- The average adult loses about two and a half quarts (about ten cups) of water each day. Therefore, drinking approximately eight to twelve cups throughout the day is sufficient.
- Heat, activity, and diet (high protein intake, caffeine, alcohol) increase your need for water.

How can you make sure you get enough water?

- Check your urine—it should be clear and light-colored.

*Dehydration: The Warning Signs*

- Nausea
- Vomiting
- Headaches
- Elevated body temperature
- Dry lips and tongue
- Dry skin
- Water retention problems
- Muscle or joint soreness
- Hoarse voice
- Constipation
- Restlessness
- Muscle cramps
- Infrequent and dark-colored urine
- Lightheadedness and loss of energy

## EXERCISE

Be as physically active as possible. For health benefits, adults should do at least two and a half hours a week of moderate-intensity or one and a quarter hours a week of vigorous intensity aerobic physical activity or an equal combination of both. You'll see a difference in your weight and your health.

Lifestyle changes that include healthy eating, regular physical activity, and maintaining a healthy weight are the keys to good health. If you need to lose weight, losing even a little will help.

Losing as little as 5 to 10 percent of your current body weight can lower your risks for many diseases.

A reasonable and safe weight loss is one to two pounds per week. It might take six months to reach your ultimate goal, but making gradual lifestyle changes can help you maintain a healthier weight for life.

*Benefits of Regular Physical Activity*

- Helps you manage your weight
- Reduces your risk of coronary heart disease
- Reduces your risk of stroke
- Decreases blood pressure
- Reduces your risk of colon cancer
- Helps prevent and control diabetes
- May decrease "bad" (LDL) cholesterol and raise "good" (HDL) cholesterol
- Helps you sleep better
- Strengthens bones and helps prevent injury

- Increases muscular strength and endurance
- Increases flexibility and range of motion
- Improves your mood
- Helps with stress and depression
- Improves self-esteem
- Makes you feel better

*Exercise Should Be FUN* So you don't like physical activity? There are lots of ways to be physically active without doing what you might consider "a workout" or "exercise."

- Go walking with others.
- Dance.
- Get the whole family involved in some physical activity like walking in a park.
- Find a beginner's exercise class that you might enjoy.
- Do housework to music.
- Try out a new sport or activity.
- Go bicycling with family or friends.
- Check out your local community center for upcoming events.
- Play golf—carry your clubs to burn more calories or use a pull-cart.

*Exercise on a Budget* Sometimes cost can be a barrier to being more physically active. There are lots of activities that involve little or no cost.

- Walking is free.
- Churches and community centers often have free events.
- Build strength using household items for weights (canned foods, small bottles of water, etc.).
- Simple stretches can improve flexibility and range of motion.
- Find a local trail.
- Buy a bicycle from a second-hand shop or at a yard sale.
- Try a new sport that doesn't require expensive equipment.
- Look at senior centers, the YMCA, and local recreational centers for free or reduced-cost activities.
- Physical activities that you build into your daily routine like taking the stairs or parking farther away and walking are free!

*Indoor Physical Activities* If the weather is bad or you prefer the indoors, there are still lots of physical activities you can do.

- Put on some music and dance.
- Do strength exercises at home using items such as water bottles and canned foods as dumbbells.

- Walk around the mall (most open early for walkers).
- Do chair stretches (ask your *MOVE!* team for a sample handout).
- Exercise to a TV program.
- Borrow an exercise video from the library or a friend (examples include chair dancing, step walking, beginner aerobics).
- Go to a gym or recreation center (join the YMCA).
- Get involved with fitness activities at a local community center or senior center.
- Too hot outside . . . take a swim at an indoor pool.
- Take a water aerobics class.
- Look for sales or visit second hand stores for used exercise equipment.
- Do indoor activities such as racquetball, tennis, roller-skating, bowling, and so on at a sports center/gym.

*Planned Physical Activities* There are lots of activities to consider if you are trying to become more active. For fitness and variety, choose activities from all three categories. Start slowly and choose activities you enjoy.

*Aerobic Activities*

- Walking
- Stair climbing
- Gardening
- Dancing—any type
- Sports
- Jogging or running
- Aerobic classes
- Roller or ice skating
- Snow skiing
- Exercise machines (treadmill, stair climber)
- Non-weight-bearing and low-impact activities (These are good for everyone but particularly beneficial for those with arthritis.)
- Swimming
- Bicycling
- Water walking or water aerobics
- Some exercise machines (stationary bike, row machine, ski machine, elliptical trainer)

*Strength Activities*

- Free weights (dumbbells, plastic bottles of water, cans of food)
- Elastic bands (available from Prosthetics)
- Conditioning exercises (e.g., sit-ups, push-ups, and pull-ups)
- Pilates

- Circuit machines
- Medicine (weighted) and balance balls

*Flexibility Activities*

- Stretching
- Chair exercises
- Yoga
- Tai Chi

## PHYSICAL ACTIVITY AND YOUR SAFETY

If you are diabetic or have heart or lung disease, check with you primary-care team before beginning a physical-activity program.

*General Safety Tips*

- Carry identification, emergency contact information, and illness information.
- Drink water before, during, and after exercise.
- Let someone know where you are going and how long you'll be gone.
- Carry a cell phone if you have one.
- Prepare for the weather.
- Wear comfortable, good-fitting socks and shoes suitable for physical activity.
- Dress to be seen. Wear bright-colored clothing. In poor light, wear safety reflective materials designed for improving your visibility to drivers.
- Use a familiar route.
- Be active in public places.
- Avoid isolated trails, paths, and poorly lit areas.
- When approaching another walker or jogger from behind, give a verbal warning before passing them.

*When to Stop Exercising* Physical activity is usually safe. Stop exercising right away if you have any of these symptoms:

- Pain, tightness, pressure, or discomfort in your chest, neck, shoulder, arm, back, or jaw
- Severe shortness of breath
- Cold sweats
- Severe nausea or vomiting
- Muscle cramps
- Trouble swallowing, talking, or seeing

- Severe headache, dizziness, or lightheadedness
- Joint pain

If symptoms don't go away after a few minutes, call 911 or go to the nearest emergency room. If the symptoms go away but return each time you exercise, see your primary-care provider.

*Increasing Physical Activity for Veterans with Physical or Medical Limitations*

*Do I need to see my health care provider before beginning a program of physical activity?*

Many veterans can begin a program of mild or moderate activity *safely* without having a check-up from their primary-care provider. Your *MOVE!* health care team can tell you whether or not you should have a check-up before starting.

In general, the following veterans should always see their provider before starting:

- Veterans with heart and/or lung conditions
- Veterans planning a program of "vigorous" activity

*What is the difference between "mild," "moderate," and "vigorous" levels of activity?*

- Mild activities should feel like slow walking/rolling. They should not cause much of a sweat or cause you to have trouble catching your breath.
- Moderate activities are like fast walking/rolling. These activities will make your heart beat a little bit faster. This may cause light sweating but should never cause you to be "out of breath" or exhausted.
- Vigorous activities will cause the heart to beat very fast. With these activities, you will sweat heavily and have some difficulty breathing.

*Are there certain activities I should avoid?*

Regardless of your limitations, very few activities are "off-limits." See the MOVE! handout, "Activity Limitations for Certain Medical Conditions."

*Will I make my condition worse by exercising?*

Physical activity almost always helps improve medical conditions. It is wise to avoid or reduce physical activity during times when your condition worsens or causes distress.

*Will my medicines affect my ability to be physically active?*

Physical activity is compatible with all medications. However, some medications require a close watch. Refer to the MOVE! handout, "Physical Activity and Medications."

*What if I'm in too much pain to be physically active?*

Regular physical activity often improves chronic pain conditions. It can sometimes take several weeks to begin to see a benefit. See your health care provider to discuss options if you feel your current pain is at a level that will keep you from even getting started with physical activity.

STAYING MOTIVATED WITH PHYSICAL ACTIVITY

Make physical activity part of your daily routine. Here are some ways to help you keep on track with your physical activity program.

- Set realistic and achievable goals.
- Schedule activity by making it part of your regular routine.
- Have a support system—friends, family, group exercise.
- Log your progress.
- Consider a trainer.
- Use music and TV fitness programs.
- Use a pedometer/odometer.
- Variety is key.
- Even small amounts of movement throughout the day add up.
- Check your progress regularly.
- Choose a convenient time of the day.
- Stay encouraged.
- Join a gym or club.
- HAVE FUN!

## *Stop Smoking*

Don't give up on quitting! No matter how long you've smoked or how many times you've tried to quit, you can be smoke-free.

Smoking is the leading preventable cause of premature death and a leading cause of illness and mortality.

Smoking and tobacco use cessation persists as one of the US Department of Veterans Affairs (VA)'s biggest public health challenges. Many veterans began using tobacco while in the military. The rate of smoking among veterans in VA health care system is higher than among the US population.

Approximately 70 percent of all smokers say they want to quit, but even the most motivated may try to quit five or six times before they are able to quit. Over three million Americans successfully quit smoking every year.

To help veterans quit smoking and tobacco use, VA offers:

- Screening for tobacco use during primary-care visits
- Individual counseling
- Prescriptions for nicotine replacement therapy, such as a nicotine patch or gum, or other medications
- Participation in evidence-based smoking cessation programs

### *Get Vaccinated and Immunized*

You can help protect yourself and others against flu and other vaccine-preventable diseases by getting immunized. Consider your lifestyle and location when deciding whether to get vaccinated against hepatitis A and B. There is no vaccine yet for hepatitis C.

#### FLU SHOTS

*Why Should I Get a Flu Shot?* Getting a flu shot is the best way to slow the spread of the flu. The flu shot can protect you against the flu.

*Who Should Get a Flu Shot?* All people age six months and older who want to reduce their risk of getting sick should get a flu shot. People more at risk of illness from the flu include:

- People with other health problems, like asthma, diabetes, and heart disease
- People older than fifty
- Women who are pregnant or want to become pregnant
- People caring for an infant or a family member with health problems
- Health care personnel

*Can I Get My Flu Shot from VA?* Veterans enrolled in VA health care and VA staff may get a flu shot at their nearest VA health care facility. If you are not enrolled in VA health care, check your eligibility online.

*Where Can My Family Members Get a Flu Shot?* VA doesn't vaccinate family members of veterans or VA staff. If your family members would like to get a flu shot, check the flu shot locator on Flu.gov.

*How Well Does the Flu Shot Work?* Studies have shown that getting the flu shot can reduce illness and death related to the flu.

*When Should I Get a Flu Shot?* Get a flu shot as soon as it becomes available in the autumn so that you are protected all winter. You will need to get a new flu shot every year to protect yourself from the most recent flu viruses. Contact your nearest VA health care facility to learn more about vaccine availability.

*How Does the Flu Shot Protect Me?* The flu shot helps your body build antibodies to fight flu viruses. These can help prevent you from getting sick with the flu. Once you get the flu shot, it takes about two weeks for your body to make enough antibodies to protect you.

*Why Do I Need a New Flu Shot Every Year?* Flu viruses can change over time. Every year, the flu shot is updated to contain the flu viruses most likely to spread that year.

*What Is in the Flu Shot?* Every year the flu shot is made of three strains of nonliving flu virus. Experts decide which strains will be in the flu shot based on the flu viruses that are spreading that year.

Sometimes the viruses change after the flu shot is made. Even if this happens, you will still get some protection from the flu shot.

*What Is the High-Dose Flu Shot?* The high-dose flu shot was approved by the federal government in 2010. It can only be given to people age sixty-five and older. It has the same three strains of flu viruses as the standard dose flu shot, but with higher doses of each.

Early studies show that the high-dose flu shot can help to build more antibodies to fight against the flu. Some people have had more discomfort at the site of the high-dose flu shot than with the standard dose flu shot. Studies are being done to learn more about the high-dose flu shot.

*Can I Get the Flu from the Flu Shot?* No. The viruses in the shot are not alive, so you cannot get the flu from the flu shot.

*Can I Still Get the Flu after I Get a Flu Shot?* Sometimes this can happen if:

- The flu shot does not contain the flu virus that is spreading.
- You are exposed to the flu before or right after getting the flu shot. You may still get the flu before the shot takes effect.
- You have a weak immune system or other illness that takes you longer to make antibodies.
- Your body fails to make antibodies after getting a flu shot.

*Is the Flu Shot Safe?* Yes, the flu shot is safe. Most people who get the flu shot have no serious side effects or allergic reactions to it. Some people may have redness or swelling on their arm where the shot was given. A very small number of people may get minor body aches, a headache, or a low-grade fever that lasts only a day or two.

The Institute of Medicine reviewed more than one thousand research articles and concluded that few health problems are associated with vaccines.

*I Am Allergic to Eggs—What Should I Do?* Recent research has found that the flu vaccine can be tolerated by people with egg allergies, without serious reactions. If you have a *severe allergy* to chicken eggs, talk with your health care provider to determine if you should get the flu shot.

*What Else Can I Do to Slow the Spread of the Flu?*

- Avoid people who are sick.
- Clean hands often.
- Keep hands away from face.
- Cover coughs and sneezes.
- Stay home when sick.

*Other Vaccinations to Consider*

*Pneumococcal:* Older people and those with certain medical conditions are most susceptible to pneumonia. People under sixty-five will need a booster shot when they reach 65 if more than five years have passed since the initial dose.

*Hepatitis A:* Recommended for those who travel to other countries or live in a US community with high rates of hepatitis A; or who have chronic liver disease, engage in male-to-male sex, or inject drugs.

*Hepatitis B:* More contagious than HIV, hepatitis B is a sexually transmitted disease than can be prevented through immunization.

*Measles, mumps, rubella (MMR):* People born after 1956 and all women of childbearing age who have not had these diseases or been vaccinated against them need to get the shots to be protected.

*Chickenpox (varicella):* Protection is necessary for those born in the United States after 1966 and have not had this disease and have not been vaccinated. Adults are at a far greater risk of complications.

*Shingles (herpes zoster):* Shingles is caused by the same virus that causes chickenpox. People who are over the age of sixty may receive a single dose of the shingles vaccine. Consult with your physician first.

*Tetanus, diphtheria (Td):* Booster doses of Td are needed at ten-year intervals.

*Vaccines for international travelers:* Many veterans and other Americans travel abroad and are likely exposed to diseases common in those countries.

## How Can Family and Friends Assist?

Make it a family goal to achieve wellness together. Be honest with each other—are you fit, are you healthy, do you eat wisely? Resolve together to adopt a wellness program that will encompass healthier eating, more exercise, and having fun. Healthier eating does not mean boring food. On the contrary, you can make wonderful meals from healthy foods. You can have fun exercising too—go for long walks, especially along the beach if you are near the coast. Adopt a rescue dog—it will provide companionship and force you to take it on walks. Take up a sport or join a club that has lots of activities out of doors. There are many ways of becoming healthier. Choose the ones that are right for you and stick to them.

## Resources Available

Aim for a Healthy Weight—National Heart Lung and Blood Institute: www.nhlbi.nih.gov

National Center for Complementary and Alternative Medicine: nccam.nih.gov/health

National Institutes of Health: www.nih.gov

NIH Senior Health: nihseniorhealth.gov/

Noise Reduction: www.noisyplanet.nidcd.nih.gov/Pages/Default.aspx

Office of Dietary Supplement: http://ods.nih.gov

Quit Smoking: Smokefree.gov

Rethinking Drinking: www.nih.gov

Weight Control—Weight-Control Information Network: win.niddk.nih.gov

Indtai's Military Community Compass Resources focus on Individual and Family Wellness for the Military Community: www.MCAeX.net to learn about education opportunities; www.MCSFeX.net to find scholarship and financial aid opportunities; www.MCJeX.net to explore job opportunities; www.MCInfoEx.net to access a one-stop knowledge base and the latest news

# References and Resource Guide


American Psychiatric Association. (1994). *Diagnostic and statistical manual of mental disorders*, 4th edition. Arlington, VA: American Psychiatric Association.

Barlow, David H. (2002). Unraveling the mysteries of anxiety and its disorders from the perspective of emotion theory. *American Psychologist* 55:1247–63.

Beck, A. T., and Steer, R. A. (2000). Beck Depression Inventory. In Task Force for the Handbook of Psychiatric Measures (Ed.), *Handbook of psychiatric measures* (pp. 519–22). Washington, DC: American Psychiatric Association.

Benedek, D. M., Ursano, R. J., Holloway, H. C., Norwood, A. E., Grieger, T. A., Engel, C. C., et al. (2001). Military and disaster psychiatry. In N. J. Smelser and P. B. Baltes (Eds.), *International encyclopedia of the social and behavioral sciences*, vol. 14 (pp. 9850–57). Oxford: Elsevier Science.

Bien, T. H., Miller, W. R., and Tonigan, J. S. (1993). Brief interventions for alcohol problems: A review. *Addiction* 88:315–35.

Briere, J. (1997). *Psychological assessment of adult posttraumatic states*. Washington, DC: American Psychological Association.

Brom, D., Kleber, R. J., and Hofman, M. C. (1993). Victims of traffic accidents: Incidence and prevention of post-traumatic stress disorder. *Journal of Clinical Psychology* 49:131–40.

Bryant, R. A., Guthrie, R. M., and Moulds, M. L. (2001). Hypnotizability in acute stress disorder. *American Journal of Psychiatry* 158:600–4.

Bryant, R. A., and Harvey, A. G. (2000). *Acute stress disorder: A handbook of theory, assessment, and treatment*. Washington, DC: American Psychological Association.

Bryant, R. A., Harvey, A. G., Dang, S. T., Sackville, T., and Basten, C. (1998). Treatment of acute stress disorder: A comparison of cognitive-behavioral therapy and supportive counseling. *Journal of Consulting and Clinical Psychology* 66:862–66.

Bryant, R. A., Sackville, T., Dang, S. T., Moulds, M., and Guthrie, R. (1999).Treating acute stress disorder: An evaluation of cognitive behavior therapy and supportive counseling techniques. *American Journal of Psychiatry* 156:1780–86.

Buss, A. H., and Durkee, A. (1957). An inventory for assessing different kinds of hostility. *Journal of Counseling Psychology* 21:343–49.

Buss, A. H., and Perry, M. (1992). The Aggression Questionnaire. *Journal of Personality and Social Psychology* 63:452–59.

Carlson, E. B. (November, 2002). Challenges to assessing traumatic stress histories in complex trauma survivors. Paper presented at the annual meeting of the International Society for Traumatic Stress Studies, Baltimore, MD.

———. (1997). Trauma assessments: A clinician's guide. New York: Guilford Press.

Carlson, E. B., and Waelde, L. (November, 2000). Preliminary psychometric properties of the Trauma Related Dissociation Scale. Paper presented at the annual meeting of the International Society for Traumatic Stress Studies, San Antonio, TX.

Chemtob, C. M., Novaco, R. W., Hamada, R. S., Gross, D. M., and Smith, G. (1997). Anger regulation deficits in combat-related posttraumatic stress disorder. *Journal of Traumatic Stress* 10:17–36.

Dawson, D. (2000). US low-risk drinking guidelines: An examination of four alternatives. *Alcoholism Clinical and Experimental Research* 24:1820–29.

DiGiovanni, C., Jr. (1999). Domestic terrorism with chemical or biological agents: Psychiatric aspects. *American Journal of Psychiatry* 156:1500–5.

Dunning, C. M. (1996). From citizen to soldier: Mobilization of reservists. In R. J. Ursano and A. E. Norwood (Eds.), *Emotional aftermath of the Persian Gulf War: Veterans, families, communities, and nations* (pp. 197–225). Washington, DC: American Psychiatric Press.

Elsayed, N. M. (1997). Toxicology of blast overpressure. *Toxicology* l 121 (1): 1–15.

Fetsch, R. J., and Jacobson, B. 2007. *Manage anger through family meetings*. Colorado State University Extension. www.ext.colostate.edu/pubs/consumer/10249.html.

Foa, E. B., Keane, T. M., and Friedman, M. J. (2000). *Effective treatments for PTSD: Practice guidelines from the International Society for Traumatic Stress Studies*. New York: Guilford.

Foa, E. B., and Rothbaum, B. O. (1998). *Treating the trauma of rape: Cognitive-behavioral therapy for PTSD*. New York: Guilford.

Franz, D.R., Jahrling, P. B., Friedlander, A. M., McClain, D. J., Hoover, D. L., Bryne, W. R., et al. (1997). Clinical recognition and management of patients exposed to biological warfare agents. *Journal of the American Medical Association* 278:399–411.

Friedman, P. D., Saitz, R., Gogineni, A., Zhang, J. X., and Stein, M. D. (2001). Validation of the screening strategy in the NIAAA—Physicians' guide to helping patients with alcohol problems. *Journal of Studies on Alcohol* 62:234–38.

Gentilello, L. M., Rivara, F. P., Donovan, D. M., Jurkovich, G. J., Daranciang, E., Dunn, et al. (1999). Alcohol interventions in a trauma center as a means of reducing the risk of injury recurrence. *Annals of Surgery* 230:473–83.

Goldman, M., Brown, S., and Christiansen, B. (2000). Alcohol Expectancy Questionnaire (AEQ). In Task Force for the Handbook of Psychiatric Measures (Ed.), *Handbook of psychiatric measures* (pp. 476–77). Washington, DC: American Psychiatric Association.

Guskiewicz, K. M., McCrea, M., Marshall S. W., Cantu, R. C., Randolph, C., Barr, W., Onate, J. A., Kelly, J. P. (2003). Cumulative effects associated with recurrent concussion in collegiate football players: The NCAA concussion study. *JAMA*, 290:2549–55.

Jones, F. D. (1995a). Disorders of frustration and loneliness. In F. D. Jones, L. R. Sparacino, V. L. Wilcox, J. M. Rothberg, and J. W. Stokes (Eds.), *War psychiatry* (pp. 63–83). Washington, DC: Borden Institute.

———. (1995b). Psychiatric principles of future warfare. In F. D. Jones, L. R. Sparacino, V. L. Wilcox, J. M. Rothberg, and J. W. Stokes (Eds.), *War psychiatry* (pp. 113–32). Washington, DC: Borden Institute.

Jordan, B. K., Marmar, C. R., Fairbank, J. A., Schlenger, W. E., Kulka, R. A., Hough, R. L., and Weiss, D. S. (1992). Problems in families of male Vietnam veterans with posttraumatic stress disorders. *Journal of Consulting and Clinical Psychology* 60:916–26.

Kelly, J. P., Nichols, J. S., Filley, C. M., Lillehie, K. O., Rubinstein, D., Kleinschmidt-DeMasters, B. K. (1991). Concussion in sports: Guidelines for the prevention of catastrophic outcome. *JAMA* 266 (20): 2867–69.

King, D. W., King, L. A., and Vogt, D. S. (2003). *Manual for the Deployment Risk and Resilience Inventory (DRRI): A collection of measures for studying deployment-related experiences in military veterans*. Boston: National Center for PTSD.

Kirkland, F. R. (1995). Postcombat reentry. In F. D. Jones, L. Sparacino, V. L. Wilcox, J. M. Rothberg, and J. W. Stokes (Eds.), *War psychiatry* (pp. 291–317). Washington, DC: Office of the Surgeon General.

Koshes, R. J. (1996). The care of those returned: Psychiatric illnesses of war. In R. J. Ursano and A. E. Norwood (Eds.), *Emotional aftermath of the Persian Gulf War: Veterans, families, communities, and nations* (pp. 393–414). Washington, DC: American Psychiatric Press.

Kubany, E. S. (1998). Cognitive therapy for trauma-related guilt. In V. M. Follette, J. I. Ruzek, and F. R. Abueg (Eds.), *Cognitive-behavioral therapies for trauma* (pp. 124–61). New York: Guilford.

Kubany, E. S., Abueg, F. R., Owens, J. A., Brennan, J. M., Kaplan, A. S., and Watson, S. B. (1995). Initial examination of a multidimensional model of trauma-related guilt: Applications to combat veterans and battered women. *Journal of Psychopathology and Behavioral Assessment* 17:353–76.

Litz, B. T. (2002). *Iraq War clinician guide*, 2nd edition. Washington, DC: U.S. Department of Defense.

Mayorga, M. A. (1997). The pathology of primary blast overpressure injury. *Toxicology* 121 (1): 17–28.

Mitchell, J. T., and Everly, G. S. (2000). Critical incident stress management and critical incident stress debriefings: Evolutions, effects and outcomes. In B. Raphael and J. P. Wilson (Eds.), *Psychological debriefing: Theory, practice, and evidence* (pp. 71–90). New York: Cambridge University Press.

Najavits, L. M. (2002). *Seeking safety: A treatment manual for PTSD and substance abuse*. New York: Guilford.

Norwood, A. E., Fullerton, C. S., and Hagen, K. P. (1996). Those left behind: military families. In R. J. Ursano and A. E. Norwood (Eds.), *Emotional aftermath of the Persian Gulf War: Veterans, families, communities, and nations* (pp. 163–96). Washington, DC: American Psychiatric Press.

Proctor, S. P., Heeren, T., White, R. F., Wolfe, J., Borgos, M. S., Davis, J. D., et al. (1998). Health status of Persian Gulf War veterans: Self-reported symptoms, environmental exposures and the effect of stress. *International Journal of Epidemiology* 27:1000–10.

Resick, P. and Schnickle, M. (1993). *Cognitive processing therapy for rape victims: A treatment manual*. Thousand Oaks, CA: Sage Publications.

Resick, P. S., and Schnicke, M. K. (2002). *Cognitive processing therapy for rape victims: A treatment manual*. Newbury Park, CA: Sage.

Resnick, H., Acierno, R., Holmes, M., Kilpatrick, D. G., and Jager, N. (1999). Prevention of post-rape psychopathology: Preliminary findings of a controlled acute rape treatment study. *Journal of Anxiety Disorders* 13 (4): 359–70.

Rothbaum, B. O., Meadows, E. A., Resick, P., and Foy, D. W. (2000). Cognitive-behavioral therapy. In E. B. Foa, T. M. Keane, and M. J. Friedman (Eds.), *Effective treatments for PTSD: Practice guidelines from the International Society for Traumatic Stress Studies* (pp. 60–83). New York: Guilford.

Ruzek, J. I. (2003). Concurrent posttraumatic stress disorder and substance use disorder among veterans: Evidence and treatment issues. In P. Ouimette and P. J. Brown (Eds.), *Trauma and substance abuse: Causes, consequences, and treatment of comorbid disorders* (pp. 191–207). Washington, DC: American Psychological Association.

Ruzek, J. I. and Zatzick, D. F. (2000). Ethical considerations in research participation among acutely injured trauma survivors: An empirical investigation. *General Hospital Psychiatry* 22 (1): 27–36.

Schlenger, W. E., Caddell, J. M., Ebert, L., Jordan, B. K., Rourke, K. M., Wilson, D., et al. (2002). Psychological reactions to terrorist attacks. Findings from the National Study of Americans' Reactions to September 11. *Journal of the American Medical Association* 288:581–88.

Scurfield, R. M., and Tice, S. (1991). Acute psycho-social intervention strategies with medical and psychiatric evacuees of "Operation Desert Storm" and their families. *Operation Desert Storm Clinician Packet*. White River Junction, VT: National Center for PTSD.

Shinseki, Eric K. (2010). Launch of homeless Intervention Program by the Department of Veteran Affairs, December 16.

Shuster, M. A., Stein, B. D., Jaycox, L. H., Collins, R. L., Marshall, G. N., Elliott, M. N., et al. (2001). A national survey of stress reactions after the September 11, 2001, terrorist attack. *New England Journal of Medicine*, 345:1507–12.

Slagle, R. A. 1985. *A family meeting handbook: Achieving family harmony happily*. Sebastopol, CA: Family Relations Foundation.

Solomon, S., Keane, T., Kaloupek, D., and Newman, E. (1996). Choosing self-report measures and structured interviews. In E. B. Carlson (Ed.), *Trauma research methodology* (pp. 56–81). Lutherville, MD: Sidran Press.

Sonnenberg, Stephen M. (1996). *The trauma of war: Stress and recovery in Vietnam veterans*. Arlington, VA: American Psychiatric Press.

Spielberger, C. D. (1988). *Manual for the State-Trait Anger Expression Inventory*. Odessa, FL: Psychological Assessment Resources.

Steil, R., and Ehlers, A. (2000). Dysfunctional meaning of posttraumatic intrusions in chronic PTSD. *Behaviour Research and Therapy* 38:537–558.

Sylvers, P., Lilenfeld, S. O., and LaPrarie, J. L., and Lilenfeld. (2011). Differences between trait fear and trait anxiety: Implications for psychopathology. *Clinical Psychology Review* 31:122–37.

Ursano, R. J., McCaughey, B. G., and Fullerton, C. S. (Eds.). (1994). *Individual and community responses to trauma and disaster: The structure of human chaos*. New York: Cambridge University Press.

U.S. Department of Veterans Affairs (2010). VA's Wide Path Out of Homelessness. See www.mentalhealth.va.gov/featureArticle_Oct-Homelessness.asp

Vlahov, D., Galea, S., Resnick, H., Boscarino, J. A., Bucuvalas, M., Gold, J., et al. (2002). Increased use of cigarettes, alcohol, and marijuana among Manhattan, New York, residents after the September 11th terrorist attacks. *American Journal of Epidemiology* 155:988–96.

Wain, H. J., and Jaccard, J. T. (1996). Psychiatric intervention with medical and surgical patients of war. In R, J. Ursano and A. E. Norwood (Eds.), *Emotional aftermath of the Persian Gulf War: Veterans, families, communities, and nations* (pp. 415–42). Washington, DC: American Psychiatric Press.

Weathers, F. W., Keane, T. M., and Davidson, J. R. T. (2001). Clinician-Administered PTSD Scale: A review of the first ten years of research. *Depression and Anxiety* 156:132–56.

Wilson, J. P., and Keane, T. M. (Eds.). (1996). *Assessing psychological trauma and PTSD*. New York: Guilford Press.

Wolfe, J. W., Keane, T. M., and Young, B. L. (1996). From soldier to civilian: Acute adjustment patterns of returned Persian Gulf veterans. In R. J. Ursano and A. E. Norwood (Eds.), *Emotional aftermath of the Persian Gulf War: Veterans, families, communities, and nations* (pp. 477–99). Washington, DC: American Psychiatric Press.

Wolfe, J., and Kimerling, R. (1997). Gender issues in the assessment of PTSD. In J. Wilson and T. M. Keane (Eds.), *Assessing psychological trauma and PTSD* (pp. 192–238). New York: Guilford.

Wright, James D., and Beth A. Rubin. (1997). Is homelessness a housing problem? In Dennis P. Culhane and Steven P. Hornburg (Eds.), *Understanding homelessness: New policy and research perspectives*. Washington, DC: Fannie Mae Foundation.

Yerkes, S. A., and Holloway, H. C. (1996). War and homecomings: The stressors of war and of returning from war. In R. J. Ursano and A. E. Norwood (Eds.), *Emotional aftermath of the Persian Gulf War: Veterans, families, communities, and nations* (pp. 25–42). Washington, DC: American Psychiatric Press.

# Glossary

**activities of daily living (ADL).** The inability to carry out activities of daily living means the inability to independently perform at least two of the six following functions: (1) bathing, (2) continence, (3) dressing, (4) eating, (5) toileting, (6) transferring in or out of a bed or chair with or without equipment.

**Air Force Assistance Fund (AFAF).** An aid organization that serves the Air Force.

**Air Force Board of Correction of Military Records (AFBCMR).** The final appeal authority for a member of the US Air Force who disagrees with the findings or disposition determination of a formal PEB that has been upheld by the SAFPC.

**Air Force Wounded Warrior (AFW2) Program.** The AFW2 Program provides personalized care and services to any airman ill or injured in support of OEF and OIF. Advocates for services on an airman's behalf, they ensure airmen have professional support and follow-up for no less than five years after separation or retirement.

**America Supports You (ASY).** America Supports You is a website that connects people, organizations, and companies to hundreds of groups that offer a variety of support to the military community.

**Americans with Disabilities Act (ADA).** Signed into law in 1990, the Americans with Disabilities Act is a civil rights law that, in many cases, prohibits discrimination based on disability.

**America's Job Bank.** America's Job Bank is a service of the US Department of Labor and the individual state employment services.

**Army Board for the Correction of Military Records (ABCMR).** The final appeal authority for a member of the US Army who disagrees with the findings or disposition determination of a formal PEB that has been upheld by the USAPDA.

**Army Career and Alumni Program (ACAP).** ACAP is a world-class transition and job assistance services program for soldiers and civilian employees and their family members.

**Army Emergency Relief (AER).** An aid organization that serves the Army.

**Army Knowledge Online (AKO).** AKO is the US Army's main intranet. It serves registered users to include active duty and retired service personnel and their family members, and provides single sign-on access to over three hundred applications and services.

**Army Wounded Warrior Program (AW2).** The program's mission is to provide personalized support for severely injured soldiers, no matter where they are located or how long their recovery takes.

**Basic Allowance for Subsistence (BAS).** A payment to members for food. Members who are hospitalized continue receiving BAS during the hospitalization.

**Board for Correction of Naval Records (BCNR).** The final appeal authority for a member of the US Navy or US Marine Corps who disagrees with the findings or disposition determination of a formal PEB that has been upheld by the DIRSECNAVCORB.

**casual pay.** Army term for an advance on a member's end of month paycheck. This payment will be automatically deducted during subsequent pay periods until paid back.

**Centers for Disease Control and Prevention (CDC).** The CDC is a government agency with the mission of promoting health and quality of life by preventing and controlling disease, injury, and disability. It is performing Vietnam veteran, Gulf War veteran, and Force Health Protections studies to evaluate the conditions of veterans as well as the care they receive.

**civilian legal counsel.** Members may hire, with their own funds, a civilian lawyer to represent them during formal PEB hearings.

**Combat-Related Injury and Rehabilitation Pay (CIP).** A monthly payment for members who were evacuated from a combat zone due to an injury. This payment was replaced by PAC, but some members who were wounded before PAC was established may be eligible for back payment of the allowance.

**Combat-Related Special Compensation (CRSC).** A monthly compensation that is intended to replace some or all of members' retired pay that is withheld due to receipt of VA compensation.

**Combat Zone Tax Exclusion (CZTE).** A policy that exempts a member from paying federal taxes while serving in an area designated as a combat zone.

**combat/operational stress injuries (COSI).** Changes in mental functioning or behavior due to the challenges of combat and its aftermath, or changes in mental functioning or behavior due to the challenges of military operations other than combat.

**combined rating.** The total percentage of disability for a member with more than one disability. This is not determined by adding percentages of disability for each condition. The formula for determining a combined rating can be found in Section 4.25 (table 1) of Title 38 of the Code of Federal Regulations.

**community-based health care organization (CBHCO).** If you are a member of the Army National Guard and Army Reserve and require only outpatient care, you may request transfer to a CBHCO. This program allows you to live at home, receive outpatient care, and perform military duties at a local military organization such as an armory or recruiting station. You cannot work at a civilian job while you are attached to a CBHCO.

**Computer/Electronic Accommodations Program (CAP).** CAP is the federal government's centrally funded accommodation program.

**Concurrent Retirement and Disability Payments (CRDP).** A program that restores retired pay on a graduated ten-year schedule for retirees with a 50 to 90 percent VA-rated disability.

**Continued Health Care Benefit Program (CHCBP).** The CHCBP is similar to but is not TRICARE. It offers temporary transitional health coverage and must be purchased within thirty days after your TRICARE eligibility ends. Benefits under CHCBP are virtually the same as those under TRS and your coverage starts the day after your separation.

**DD Form 214—Certificate of Release or Discharge from Active Duty.** The Report of Separation contains information normally needed to verify military service for benefits, retirement, employment, and membership in veterans' organizations.

**DD Form 2586—Verification of Military Experience and Training.** The DD Form 2586 is created from a service member's automated records on file. It lists military job experience and training history, recommended college credit information, and civilian-equivalent job titles. This document is designed to help the member apply for jobs, but it is not a résumé.

**DD Form 2648 Pre-separation Counseling Checklist.** A form used by the DoD that helps Transition Assistance Program employees assist members in transitioning out of the military and into civilian life.

**Department of Veterans Affairs (VA).** The federal agency responsible for providing a broad range of programs and services to service members and veterans as required by Title 38 of the US Code.

**Director, Secretary of the Navy Council of Review Boards (DIRSECNAVCORB).** The governing body for the US Navy overseeing the DES process for the service. A sailor or marine may appeal a PEB finding with the DIRSECNAVCORB, which has the authority to uphold the PEB findings, issue revised findings, or send the case back to the PEB for another review.

**Disability Evaluation System (DES).** A system or process of the US government for evaluating the nature and extent of disabilities affecting members of the armed forces; it includes medical/psychological evaluations, physical evaluations, counseling of members, and mechanisms for the final disposition of disability determinations.

**Disability Evaluation System (DES) Pilot.** A joint DoD-VA Disability Evaluation System Pilot was begun in the National Capital Region in November 2007 to improve the timeliness, effectiveness, and transparency of the DES review process. Under the pilot, VA performs one medical exam and rates a member's disabilities. This examination and rating is used by the PEB to determine fitness for duty and disposition, and by VA to determine VA disability compensation.

**disability retirement pay.** The monthly allowance paid to members who are placed on the TDRL or PDRL. The formula for determining the amount of disability retirement pay is found in chapter 9.

**Disabled Transition Assistance Program (DTAP).** DTAP works with members who may be released because of a disability or who believe they have a disability qualifying them for VA's Vocational Rehabilitation and Employment Program (VR&E). The goal of DTAP is to encourage and assist potentially eligible service members in making an informed decision about VA's VR&E program. It is also intended to quickly deliver vocational-rehabilitation services to eligible service members by assisting them in filing an application for vocational-rehabilitation benefits.

**Disabled Veterans Outreach Program (DVOP) Specialists.** A Department of Labor employee trained to help veterans make the important adjustment to the civilian job market.

**DoD Job Search.** A website that is a part of the America's Job Bank service designed solely for service members.

**DoD Suicide Prevention and Risk Reduction Committee's (SPARRC) Preventing Suicide Network.** The DoD SPARRC Preventing Suicide Network is a resource center aimed at providing authoritative and problem-specific information about suicide prevention.

**efficiency.** Efficiency is the measure of a member's total health minus his or her disability. A member with a 60 percent disability has only 40 percent of his or her total health that is not impacted by the disability.

**Family and Medical Leave Act (FMLA).** The federal law that provides unpaid leave and job protection to those who have family members with medical conditions that require their presence. The Fiscal Year 2008 National Defense Authorization Act authorized the expansion of the FMLA to support families of recovering service members.

**Family Liaison Officer (FLO).** An Air Force employee appointed to every airman with a combat-related injury to assist in providing support to the recovering airman's family.

**Family Separation Allowance (FSA).** Pay a member receives if he or she has dependents and is away from his or her permanent duty station for more than thirty days for temporary duty or on a temporary change of station, to include a deployment.

**fit/unfit.** Finding of the PEB. Fitness or unfitness is solely determined by the ability of the member to perform the duties of his or her office, grade, rank, or rating because of disease or injury.

**formal Physical Evaluation Board (PEB).** If a member disagrees with the informal PEB findings or disposition, he or she may request a formal PEB, appear before the board in person, obtain military or civilian legal counsel to represent him or her, call witnesses, present evidence, and present testimony on his or her own behalf.

**GL-2005.261—Traumatic Injury Protection Payment.** The form used to request insurance payment for service-connected traumatic injury or loss from service in OIF/OEF.

**Hardship Duty Pay Location (HDP-L).** Pay a member receives while serving in a location that the Secretary of Defense identifies as a hardship duty location.

**Health and Human Services (HHS).** HHS is the principal agency for protecting the health of all Americans and providing essential human services, especially for those who are least able to help themselves.

**Health Resources and Service Administration (HRSA).** HRSA is the primary federal agency for improving access to health care services for people who are uninsured, isolated, or medically vulnerable.

**hemiplegia.** Paralysis affecting only one side of the body.

**hospitalized.** For the purposes of some pay entitlements, members are considered hospitalized if they were admitted as an inpatient or were receiving extensive rehabilitation as an outpatient while living in quarters affiliated with the military health care system.

**Hostile Fire Pay/Imminent Danger Pay (HFP/IDP).** Pay a member receives while serving in an area the president identifies as placing him or her in imminent danger or that he or she may come under hostile fire.

**Individual Transition Plan (ITP).** The ITP is a framework a member can use to fulfill realistic career goals based upon his or her unique skills, knowledge, experience, and abilities. The ITP identifies actions and activities associated with a member's transition.

**informal Physical Evaluation Board.** The initial meeting of a PEB to determine a disposition of the member's medical case. The member will not be present at the informal PEB. The informal PEB will determine fit/unfit and the member's disposition based on the member's case file. The PEBLO counsels the member on the findings of the informal PEB and provides options for appeal of those findings.

**Invitational Travel Authorizations (ITAs), Invitational Travel Orders (ITOs), or Emergency Family Member Travel (EFMT).** Military travel orders that allow a recovering service member's family to travel and stay with him or her during treatment and recovery after suffering a wound, illness, or injury.

**Job Accommodation Network (JAN).** A free service from the Department of Labor's Office of Disability Employment Policy that provides personalized worksite accommodations, information regarding the ADA and other disability-related information, and information about self-employment.

**local veterans employment representative (LVER).** A Department of Labor employee trained to help veterans make the important adjustment to the civilian job market.

**Medical Evaluation Board (MEB).** A board, generally comprising medical officers, that determines if a member meets medical retention standards for his or her service. The board may recommend a return to duty or send the member's case to a Physical Evaluation Board.

**MedlinePlus.** MedlinePlus is a service of the US National Library of Medicine and the National Institutes of Health that provides resources regarding all aspects of veterans' health including recent news, treatments, rehabilitation and recovery programs, condition-specific information, financial issues, as well as ongoing clinical trials and research.

**mild traumatic brain injury (mTBI).** Mild traumatic brain injury (concussion) is caused by blunt trauma to the head or acceleration/deceleration forces jogging the brain within the skull, which may or may not produce a period of unconsciousness. Mild TBI is defined as an injury to the brain as a result of any period of observed or self-reported confusion, disorientation, or impaired consciousness; dysfunction of memory around the time of injury (amnesia); or loss of consciousness lasting less than thirty minutes. No other obvious neurological deficits or intracranial complications (e.g., hematoma/blood clot) should be found, and normal computed tomography (CT) findings should be present.

**Military Severely Injured Center (MSIC).** A DoD call-in support program that provides information regarding medical care and rehabilitation;

education, training, and job placement; personal mobility and functioning; accommodations; counseling; and financial resources.

**minority opinion.** When a member of the PEB disagrees with the findings of the board, he or she will write a minority opinion outlining the areas of disagreement that becomes part of the board findings.

**Montgomery G.I. Bill (MGIB).** The MGIB provides up to thirty-six months of education benefits to eligible veterans for college, technical, or vocational courses; correspondence courses; apprenticeship/job training; flight training; high-tech training; licensing and certification tests; entrepreneurship training; and certain entrance examinations.

**Montgomery G.I. Bill—Selected Reserve (MGIB-SR).** The MGIB-SR program may be available to you if you are a member of the Selected Reserve. The Selected Reserve includes the Army Reserve, Navy Reserve, Air Force Reserve, Marine Corps Reserve, and Coast Guard Reserve, and the Army National Guard and the Air National Guard. You may use this education-assistance program for degree programs, certificate or correspondence courses, cooperative training, independent study programs, apprenticeship/on-the-job training, and vocational flight-training programs.

**National Association for People of Color Against Suicide (NOPCAS).** NOPCAS is a nonprofit organization with the goal of stopping suicide in minority communities.

**National Association of Child Care Resource and Referral Agencies (NACCRRA).** NACCRRA is an organization through which a service member can get assistance to find and pay for safe, licensed child care services for a period of six months during his or her recuperation.

**National Capital Region (NCR).** Washington, D.C. and the surrounding areas.

**National Defense Authorization Act for Fiscal Year 2008 (NDAA).** Public Law 110-181 that authorizes expenditures and provides guidance for the federal government concerning national defense. In the Fiscal Year 2008 version, a large section was devoted to wounded warrior issues.

**National Institute of Diabetes, Digestive and Kidney Diseases (NIDDK).** NIDDK supports twenty-two research projects related to veterans of military service.

**National Institute of Mental Health (NIMH).** NIMH conducts projects on trauma and post-traumatic stress disorder that involve veteran populations.

**National Institute on Deafness and Other Communicative Disorders (NIDCD).** The NIDCD studies the molecular mechanisms that cause the loss of hearing from exposure to loud noise.

**National Institute on Dental and Craniofacial Research (NIDCR).** The NIDCR conducts ongoing research in tissue engineering and regeneration for wounds to the head and face.

**National Strategy for Suicide Prevention (NSSP).** The NSSP is a collaborative effort between SAMSHA, CDC, NIH, HRSA, and HHS and provides facts about suicide, recent publications, and resources designed to spread knowledge of the seriousness of suicides.

**Navy Marine Corps Relief Society (NMCRS).** An aid organization that serves the Navy and Marine Corps.

**Navy Safe Harbor.** The Navy Safe Harbor program provides personalized assistance to severely injured sailors and their families.

**ombudsman.** An ombudsman is assigned to or near a major military facility or VA medical facility to further assist in the transition by helping service members connect with local agencies and community groups.

**Operation Enduring Freedom (OEF).** OEF includes casualties that occurred in and around Afghanistan: in Afghanistan, Pakistan, and Uzbekistan. Other locations: in Guantanamo Bay (Cuba), Djibouti, Eritrea, Ethiopia, Jordan, Kenya, Kyrgyzstan, Philippines, Seychelles, Sudan, Tajikistan, Turkey, and Yemen.

**Operation Iraqi Freedom (OIF).** OIF includes casualties that occurred on or after March 19, 2003, in the Arabian Sea, Bahrain, Gulf of Aden, Gulf of Oman, Iraq, Kuwait, Oman, Persian Gulf, Qatar, Red Sea, Saudi Arabia, and United Arab Emirates. Prior to March 19, 2003, casualties in these countries were considered OEF.

**paraplegia.** Complete paralysis of the lower half of the body including both legs, usually caused by damage to the spinal cord.

**partial pay.** Air Force term for an advance on a member's end of month paycheck. This payment will be automatically deducted during subsequent pay periods until paid back.

**Patient Administration Team (PAT).** A nonmedical care organization that assists members of the military in issues related to their hospitalization and recovery.

**Pay and Allowance Continuation (PAC).** A new policy allowing members evacuated from a combat zone to continue receiving all combat pay and allowances they received prior to the injury for the first year they are hospitalized.

**per diem.** A daily allowance paid to a person on military travel orders to cover food, lodging, and incidentals. In cases where lodging or food is provided by the government, this payment will only be for the $3.50 incidental rate.

**Permanent Disabled Retirement List (PDRL).** PEB disposition finding for a member who has one or more service unfitting condition(s) with a combined rating of 30 percent or higher, was incurred in the line of duty, and is considered stable. This disposition also covers members who have served twenty or more years, have one or more service unfitting condition(s) with a combined rating of 20 percent or less, was incurred in the line of duty, and are considered stable.

**Personnel Service Detachment (PSD).** A military personnel office that assists members and their families with pay and personnel problems.

**Physical Evaluation Board (PEB).** A board, generally comprising a senior line officer, senior personnel officer, and senior medical officer, that determines if a member is fit or unfit for continued service. This board may recommend a return to duty, separation with or without benefits, or medical retirement (temporary or permanent).

**Physical Evaluation Board Disposition.** The findings of a PEB on a member's medical case. Member can be found fit and returned to duty, found unfit and separated with or without benefits, or medically retired on either the Permanent or Temporary Disability Retirement List.

**Physical Evaluation Board Liaison Officer (PEBLO).** The person assigned to assist the service member through the DES process. Duties include counseling the member on the process as well as building the case file used by the PEB to determine fitness for duty.

**Post-9/11 GI Bill.** Post-9/11 GI Bill is a new benefit providing educational assistance to individuals who have served on active duty on or after September 11, 2001. It provides additional monetary benefits for members, including a housing and book allowance, and is limited by the cost of the highest public school tuition costs in the state the member resides, rather than a set cap like in the Montgomery GI Bill. It also allows for transfer of benefits to family members in certain instances.

**post-traumatic stress disorder (PTSD).** A traumatic stress injury that fails to heal such that the symptoms and behaviors it causes remain significantly troubling or disabling beyond thirty days after their onset.

**Project Action.** Project Action maintains a national paratransit database.

**quadriplegia**. Paralysis of all four limbs.

**REALifelines.** A Department of Labor program to help injured veterans return to fulfilling, productive civilian lives using federal, state, and local level efforts to create a network of resources that focus on veteran well-being and job-placement assistance.

**Recovery Coordinator.** A person assigned to make sure your needs are being met by the right person in the right place and on time.

**Recovery Plan.** The Recovery Coordinator prepares a Recovery Plan that lays out the path for you to meet personal and professional goals.

**respite care.** Respite care includes adult day-care and home-care services, as well as overnight stays in a facility, and can be provided a few hours a week or for a weekend.

**return to duty.** PEB disposition finding for a member who does not have a service unfitting condition.

**Savings Deposit Program (SDP).** Members deployed to combat zones may put up to $10,000 of their pay in this program and earn 10 percent interest on the money deposited.

**Secretary of the Air Force Personnel Council (SAFPC).** Organization that can uphold a PEB finding, revise the findings of a PEB, or return the case to the PEB for further review. Airmen may present a written rebuttal to the SAFPC if they disagree with the PEB findings.

**separate with severance pay.** The PEB disposition finding for a member who has a service unfitting condition, but whose combined rating is 20 percent or less.

**separate without benefits.** The PEB disposition finding for a member who has a service unfitting condition, but whose condition is not found to be in the line of duty, or is found to have existed before entry into service and not aggravated by service.

**Servicemembers' Group Life Insurance (SGLI).** SGLI is a program of low-cost group life insurance for service members on active duty, ready reservists, members of the National Guard, members of the Commissioned Corps of the National Oceanic and Atmospheric Administration and the Public Health Service, cadets and midshipmen of the four service academies, and members of the Reserve Officer Training Corps.

**severance pay.** A one-time, lump-sum payment for members separated from the military for medical reasons, but who receive a combined rating of 20 percent or less for unfitting conditions. The formula for determining the amount of service pay a member will receive is found in chapter 9.

**SGLV 8714—Veterans Group Life Insurance (VGLI).** The form used to convert SGLI to VGLI.

**SGLV 8715—SGLI Disability Extension.** The form used to request an extension of the SGLI coverage for two years from date of discharge from the military for those who are totally disabled.

**Small Business Administration (SBA) loans.** Business loans are available to veterans through programs of the SBA. In addition, SBA offers loans specifically to Vietnam-era and disabled veterans.

**Social Security Administration (SSA).** The SSA is the government agency that is charged with ensuring the economic security of Americans. While you work you pay taxes into the Social Security system, and when you retire or become disabled, you, your spouse, and your dependent children receive monthly benefits that are based on your reported earnings. Also, your survivors can collect benefits if you die.

**Social Security Disability Insurance Program (SSDI).** SSDI pays benefits to you and certain members of your family if you are "insured" meaning that you worked long enough and paid Social Security taxes.

**special pay.** Navy / Marine Corps term for an advance on a member's end of month paycheck. This payment will be automatically deducted during subsequent pay periods until paid back.

**stable.** A condition that, in the doctor's opinion, is unlikely to improve to the point a member can return to duty.

**Substance Abuse and Mental Health Services Administration (SAMHSA).** SAMHSA is an agency within the DHHS that focuses on building resilience and facilitating recovery for people with or at risk for mental or substance-use disorders.

**Suicide Awareness Voices of Education (SAVE).** SAVE is a nonprofit organization with the goal of preventing suicide through public awareness and education, reducing stigma, and serving as a resource to those touched by suicide.

**Supplemental Security Income (SSI).** SSI is a federal income-supplement program funded by general tax revenues (not Social Security taxes). It is designed to help aged, blind, and disabled people who have little or no income and provides cash to meet basic needs for food, clothing, and shelter.

**Temporary Disability Retirement List (TDRL).** The PEB disposition finding for a member who has one or more service unfitting condition(s) with a combined rating of 30 percent or higher, was incurred in the line of duty, and is not considered stable.

**Transition Assistance Program (TAP).** TAP is a program designed to ease the transition from military service to the civilian workforce and community.

**traumatic brain injury (TBI).** Traumatic brain injury is a neurological injury with possible physical, cognitive, behavioral, and emotional symptoms. Like all injuries, TBI is most appropriately and accurately diagnosed as soon as possible after the injury. TBI is not a mental health condition. The range of TBI includes mild, moderate, severe, and penetrating. Well after the injury event, service personnel may have residual symptoms from a TBI and new or emerging PTSD symptoms. If the TBI has not been previously identified or documented, an accurate description of the traumatic events in theater usually allows a well-trained clinician to make a distinction between TBI and PTSD or other mental health conditions.

**traumatic event.** A qualifying traumatic injury is an injury or loss caused by application of external force or violence (a traumatic event) *or* a condition whose cause can be directly linked to a traumatic event.

**traumatic injury.** Traumatic injury is derived by external force or violence or a condition that can be linked to a traumatic event.

**Traumatic Service members' Group Life Insurance (TSGLI).** An insurance program related to the Service members' Group Life Insurance that pays a member who has suffered a severe loss, such as a leg or arm amputation.

**TRICARE.** The military medical health care system.

**TRICARE Dental Program (TDP).** The dental insurance coverage offered to those who are TRICARE eligible.

**TRICARE Online.** TRICARE Online is the entry point that offers beneficiaries access to available health care services, benefits, and information.

**TRICARE Reserve Select (TRS).** TRS is a premium-based plan that you purchase. You may receive care from any TRICARE-authorized provider without a referral. Referrals are not required, but some medical services will require prior authorization. For information or assistance with qualifying for and purchasing TRS, check the TRICARE website.

**Troops to Teachers (TTT).** The TTT program is funded and overseen by the Department of Education and operated by the DoD. The TTT program helps recruit quality teachers for schools that serve students from low income families throughout America.

**US Air Force Physical Disability Division.** Processing agency for all formal and informal PEB cases in the US Air Force. This organization reviews all PEB findings and dispositions, referring those it feels need further review to the Secretary of the Air Force Personnel Council.

**US Army Physical Disability Agency (USAPDA).** The governing body for the US Army overseeing the DES process for the service. All PEB findings are sent to the USAPDA, and 20 percent of the cases are randomly reviewed for quality assurance purposes. Any case with a minority opinion will be automatically reviewed. Soldiers may appeal a PEB finding with the USAPDA, which has the authority to uphold the PEB findings, issue revised findings, or send the case back to the PEB for another review.

**US Public Health Service (USPHS).** "Healthier Vets," the Surgeon General's joint DHHS-VA initiative, is designed to help veterans and their families remain physically active after they have separated from the military.

**unemployment compensation for ex-service members.** Service members separating from active duty may qualify for unemployment compensation if they are unable to find a new job.

**VA Form 10-8678—Clothing Allowance.** The form used to apply for a clothing allowance if a service-connected disability requiring a prosthetic device or orthopedic appliance (such as a wheelchair) leads to damage to a veteran's clothes.

**VA Form 21-4502—Vehicle Purchase and Adaptation.** The form used to apply for a one-time grant toward the purchase of a vehicle with adaptive equipment approved by VA for a veteran or service member with certain disabilities.

**VA Form 21-526—Compensation and Pension.** The form used to request VA provide service-related disability compensation, or a pension for those who are wartime veterans with non-service-connected disabilities.

**VA Form 21-8940—Increased Compensation Based on Unemployability.** The form used to request compensation based on an inability to work due to total disability from service-connected disability(s).

**VA Form 22-1990—VA Education Benefits.** The form used to apply for multiple education benefits, including the Montgomery GI Bill Educational Assistance Program; Montgomery GI Bill Selected Reserve Educational Assistance Program; Reserve Educational Assistance Program; Post-Vietnam-Era Veterans Educational Assistance Program; National Call to Serve Program; and the Transfer of Entitlement Program.

**VA Form 22-5490—Survivors' and Dependents' Educational Assistance.** The form used to apply for educational assistance to a spouse or child if the member is permanently and totally disabled as a result of a service-connected disability, dies of a service-connected disability, or while rated permanently and totally disabled, or is missing in action or a prisoner of war.

**VA Form 26-4555—Housing Adaptation.** The form used to apply for grants for constructing an adapted home or modifying an existing home to meet a disabled veteran/service member's needs.

**VA Form 28-1900—Disabled Veterans Application for Vocational Rehabilitation.** Form used to apply for vocational rehabilitation and employment benefits.

**VA Form 28-8832—Application for Counseling.** The form used to apply for vocational and educational counseling.

**VA Form 29-0188—Application for Supplemental Service-Disabled Veterans (RH) Life Insurance.** The form used to apply for Supplemental Service-Disabled Veterans Insurance.

**VA Form 29-357—Claim for Disability Insurance Benefits.** The form used to apply for waiver of premiums on a Service-Disabled Veterans Insurance policy.

**VA Form 29-4364—Application for Service-Disabled Veterans Life Insurance.** The form used to apply for Service-Disabled Veterans Insurance (S-DVI).

**VA Form 29-8636—Veterans Mortgage Life Insurance Statement.** The form used to apply for Veterans Mortgage Life Insurance (VMLI).

**VA Schedule for Rating Disabilities (VASRD).** The document used to determine the severity of a member's disability expressed as a percentage of disability.

**Vet Center Program.** Vet centers, run by VA, provide free individual, group, and family counseling to all veterans who served in any combat zone.

**Veterans Educational Assistance Program (VEAP).** VEAP is available if you elected to make contributions from your military pay to participate in this education benefit program. You may use these benefits for degree, certificate, correspondence, apprenticeship / on-the-job training programs, and vocational flight-training programs. In certain circumstances, remedial, deficiency, and refresher training may also be available. Benefit entitlement is one to thirty-six months depending on the number of monthly contributions. You have ten years from your release from active duty to use VEAP benefits. If there is entitlement not used after the ten-year period, your portion remaining in the fund will be automatically refunded.

**Veterans Preference (federal hiring).** Veterans who are disabled, served on active duty in the military during certain specified time periods, or in military campaigns, are entitled to preference over others in hiring for virtually all federal government jobs.

**Veterans Upward Bound (VUB) program.** The VUB program is a free Department of Education program designed to help eligible US military veterans refresh their academic skills so that they can successfully complete the postsecondary school of their choosing.

**Veterans Service Organization (VSO).** Organizations that are chartered by Congress and / or recognized by VA for claims representation for today's returning service members, veterans, and their families.

**Vocational Rehabilitation and Employment (VR&E).** VR&E delivers timely and effective vocational rehabilitation services to veterans with service-connected disabilities and to certain service members awaiting discharge due to a medical condition.

**Wounded Warrior Pay Management Team (WWPMT).** Highly trained finance experts who the Defense Finance and Accounting Service have prepared to deal with the complex issues surrounding pay and allowances for recovering service members.

**Wounded Warrior Project (WWP).** A project offering programs and services to severely injured members during the time of active duty through transition to civilian life.

**Wounded Warrior Regiment/Marine for Life Injured Support.** The program is to "provide information, advocacy and assistance to injured Marines, Sailors injured while serving with Marines, and their families, in order to minimize the difficulties and worries they face as they navigate the stressful and confusing process."

# Index

# About the Authors

**Cheryl Lawhorne-Scott** is a clinical therapist with an eighteen-year track record of counseling services specializing in trauma care, post-traumatic stress, and traumatic brain-injury treatment for wounded, ill, and injured service members and their families. As a senior consultant, under the Office of the Secretary of Defense, she is part of a team that seeks innovative and proactive ways to enhance resources and services to military members and their families. She recently participated in the corporate mission, vision, and implementation of projects for the Department of Defense to align current and future strategic plans and objectives. She possesses proven expertise in both program management and clinical experts in research, business development, and wounded care. Proud spouse and teammate to Lt. Col. Jeff Scott, and mom to Evan and Quinn.

**Don Philpott** is editor of *International Homeland Security Journal* and has been writing, reporting, and broadcasting on international events, trouble spots, and major news stories for almost forty years. For twenty years he was a senior correspondent with Press Association-Reuters, the wire service, and traveled the world on assignments including Northern Ireland, Lebanon, Israel, South Africa, and Asia.

He writes for magazines and newspapers in the United States and Europe and is a regular contributor to radio and television programs on security and other issues. He is the author of more than 120 books on a wide range of subjects and has had more than five thousand articles printed in publications around the world. His recent books include the *Military Life* series, *Terror—Is America Safe?*, *Workplace Violence Prevention*, and the *Education Facility Security Handbook*.